S0-EJH-999

PROGRESS IN CLINICAL AND BIOLOGICAL RESEARCH

Series Editors

Nathan Back
George J. Brewer
Vincent P. Eijsvoogel
Robert Grover

Kurt Hirschhorn
Seymour S. Kety
Sidney Udenfriend
Jonathan W. Uhr

1983 TITLES

Vol 115: **Prevention of Hereditary Large Bowel Cancer,** John R.F. Ingall, Anthony J. Mastromarino, *Editors*

Vol 116: **New Concepts in Thyroid Disease,** Roberto J. Soto, Gerardo Sartorio, Ismael de Forteza, *Editors*

Vol 117: **Reproductive Toxicology,** Donald R. Mattison, *Editor*

Vol 118: **Growth and Trophic Factors,** J. Regino Perez-Polo, Jean de Vellis, Bernard Haber, *Editors*

Vol 119: **Oncogenes and Retroviruses: Evaluation of Basic Findings and Clinical Potential,** Timothy E. O'Connor, Frank J. Rauscher, Jr., *Editors*

Vol 120: **Advances in Cancer Control: Research and Development,** Paul F. Engstrom, Paul N. Anderson, Lee E. Mortenson, *Editors*

Vol 121: **Progress in Cancer Control III: A Regional Approach,** Curtis Mettlin, Gerald P. Murphy, *Editors*

Vol 122: **Advances in Blood Substitute Research,** Robert B. Bolin, Robert P. Geyer, George Nemo, *Editors*

Vol 123: **California Serogroup Viruses,** Charles H. Calisher, Wayne H. Thompson, *Editors*

Vol 124: **Epilepsy: An Update on Research and Therapy,** Giuseppe Nisticò, Raoul Di Perri, H. Meinardi, *Editors*

Vol 125: **Sulfur Amino Acids: Biochemical and Clinical Aspects,** Kinya Kuriyama, Ryan J. Huxtable, and Heitaroh Iwata, *Editors*

Vol 126: **Membrane Biophysics II: Physical Methods in the Study of Epithelia,** Mumtaz A. Dinno, Arthur B, Callahan, Thomas C. Rozzell, *Editors*

Vol 127: **Orphan Drugs and Orphan Diseases: Clinical Realities and Public Policy,** George J. Brewer, *Editor*

Vol 128: **Research Ethics,** Kåre Berg, Knut Erik Tranøy, *Editors*

Vol 129: **Zinc Deficiency in Human Subjects,** Ananda S. Prasad, Ayhan O. Çavdar, George J. Brewer, Peter J. Aggett, *Editors*

Vol 130: **Progress in Cancer Control IV: Research in the Cancer Center,** Curtis Mettlin and Gerald P. Murphy, *Editors*

Vol 131: **Ethopharmacology: Primate Models of Neuropsychiatric Disorders,** Klaus A. Miczek, *Editor*

Vol 132: **13th International Cancer Congress,** Edwin A. Mirand, William B. Hutchinson, and Enrico Mihich, *Editors.* Published in 5 Volumes: Part A: **Current Perspectives in Cancer.** Part B: **Biology of Cancer (1).** Part C: **Biology of Cancer (2).** Part D: **Research and Treatment.** Part E: **Cancer Management**

Vol 133: **Non-HLA Antigens in Health, Aging, and Malignancy,** Elias Cohen and Dharam P. Singal, *Editors*

Please see pages following the index for previous titles in this series

13th International Cancer Congress, Part A

CURRENT PERSPECTIVES IN CANCER

⌊International Cancer Congress (13th : 1982 : Seattle, Wash.)

13th International Cancer Congress, Part A

CURRENT PERSPECTIVES IN CANCER

**Proceedings of the 13th International Cancer Congress
September 8–15, 1982
Seattle, Washington**

Editors

Edwin A. Mirand
Roswell Park Memorial Institute
Buffalo, New York

William B. Hutchinson
Fred Hutchinson Cancer Research Center
Seattle, Washington

Enrico Mihich
Roswell Park Memorial Institute
Buffalo, New York

ALAN R. LISS, INC. • NEW YORK

RC 261
A 1
I 55
v. 1
1982

Address all Inquiries to the Publisher
Alan R. Liss, Inc., 150 Fifth Avenue, New York, NY 10011

Copyright © 1983 Alan R. Liss, Inc.

Printed in the United States of America.

Under the conditions stated below the owner of copyright for this book hereby grants permission to users to make photocopy reproductions of any part or all of its contents for personal or internal organizational use, or for personal or internal use of specific clients. This consent is given on the condition that the copier pay the stated per-copy fee through the Copyright Clearance Center, Incorporated, 21 Congress Street, Salem, MA 01970, as listed in the most current issue of "Permissions to Photocopy" (Publisher's Fee List, distributed by CCC, Inc.), for copying beyond that permitted by sections 107 or 108 of the US Copyright Law. This consent does not extend to other kinds of copying, such as copying for general distribution, for advertising or promotional purposes, for creating new collective works, or for resale.

Library of Congress Cataloging in Publication Data

International Cancer Congress (13th : 1982 : Seattle, Wash.)
13th International Cancer Congress.

(Progress in clinical and biological research ; 132)
Includes bibliographies and indexes.
Contents: pt. A. Current perspectives in cancer -- pt. B. Biology of cancer (1) -- pt. C. Biology of cancer (2) -- pt. D. Research and treatment -- pt. E. Cancer management.
1. Cancer--Congresses. I. Mirand, Edwin A., 1926–   . II. Hutchinson, William B. III. Mihich, Enrico. IV. Title. V. Title: Thirteenth International Cancer Congress. VI. Series. [DNLM: 1. Medical oncology--Congresses. W1 PR668E v.132 / QZ 200 I604 1982z]
RC261.A2I56 1982a   616.99′4   83-48399
ISBN 0-8451-0132-3 (set)
ISBN 0-8451-0174-9 (pt. A)

Contents

Contributors   ix

Foreword
Edwin A. Mirand   xi

Preface to Part A
Edwin A. Mirand   xiii

PLENARY CONGRESS LECTURES

The Role of National Efforts in Developing Coordinated Programs
on International Oncology
Gerald P. Murphy   3

The Role of Organization in Cancer Control
Francis J. Wilcox   25

Why Surgical Oncology?
Harold O. Douglass, Jr.   31

Advances in Cancer Therapeutics: Chemotherapy
Vincent T. DeVita, Jr.   47

Cancer Epidemiology: Past, Present, and Future
C.S. Muir   71

Recent Progress in Radiation Oncology
Maurice Tubiana   107

The Role of Intensive Chemoradiotherapy and Marrow
Transplantation in the Treatment of Disseminated Malignant
Disease
E. Donnall Thomas   133

Biology and Oncology: Regulation of Growth, Differentiation and
Malignancy
Leo Sachs   141

FINAL CONGRESS REPORT

Edwin A. Mirand   145

INDEX   209

Contributors

Vincent T. DeVita, Jr., National Cancer Institute, Bethesda, MD **[47]**

Harold O. Douglass, Jr., Department of Surgical Oncology, Roswell Park Memorial Institute, Buffalo, NY **[31]**

Edwin A. Mirand, Roswell Park Memorial Institute, Buffalo, NY **[145]**

C.S. Muir, Descriptive Epidemiology Unit, International Agency for Research on Cancer, Lyon Cedex, France **[71]**

Gerald P. Murphy, Roswell Park Memorial Institute, Buffalo, NY **[3]**

Leo Sachs, Department of Genetics, Weizmann Institute of Science, Rehovot, Israel **[141]**

Maurice Tubiana, Institut Gustave-Roussy, Villejuif, France **[107]**

E. Donnall Thomas, University of Washington School of Medicine, Fred Hutchinson Cancer Research Center, Seattle, WA **[133]**

Francis J. Wilcox, American Cancer Society, Eau Claire, WI **[25]**

The number in brackets is the opening page number of the contributor's article.

Foreword

The papers presented in the Plenary Lectures and the Congress Symposia at the 13th International Cancer Congress, September 8–15, 1982, Seattle, Washington, are included in these volumes. The United States was the official host of the Congress, which was held under the auspices of the International Union Against Cancer (UICC), and the Fred Hutchinson Cancer Research Center, Seattle, Washington was the host institution.

Dr. William B. Hutchinson of the Fred Hutchinson Cancer Research Center was the Congress President and Dr. Edwin A. Mirand of Roswell Park Memorial Institute, Buffalo, New York, was the Secretary-General.

The scientific program of the Congress contained over 4,000 presentations. The National Program Committee, chaired by Dr. Enrico Mihich of Roswell Park Memorial Institute, felt that it would be appropriate to include only the papers from the Plenary Lectures and the Congress Symposia to keep the number of volumes at a reasonable level. These papers are presented in five volumes.

Volume A — Final Report of the Secretary-General that includes the organizational details of the scientific program

                — Plenary Lectures

Volumes B & C — Basic science topics in oncology

Volumes D & E — Clinical oncology topics

Since it would be impossible to cover all the areas of oncology presented at the Congress, by presenting the plenary and symposia sessions, we attempted to select the most rapidly advancing and promising areas of clinical and basic research. A good index of the growth in the field of oncology can be obtained by comparing the publications of this meeting with the last cancer congress publications (12th International Cancer Congress) held in Buenos Aires from October 5–10, 1978.

Looking over the topics covered herein, one can only marvel at the tremendous rate of progress and the increase in interest in oncology in the past four years. This reflects the developments in molecular biology as it relates to cancer viral and chemical carcinogenesis, in the design and evaluation of clinical trials, biological response modifiers, cancer nursing, psychosocial aspects of cancer, etc.

On behalf of the Congress officers, we wish to express our gratitude to the National Program Committee and to all the scientists, physicians, dentists, nurses, and other participants engaged in oncology who attended this Congress and who made it a success. I am sure that both the scientific and social interchange which was experienced at the Seattle meeting will have a positive, lasting effect on our lives. We hope to see you at the 14th International Cancer Congress to be held in Budapest, Hungary in 1986 to further the scientific and social interaction.

The editors are deeply indebted to all the authors for their outstanding contributions to these volumes.

We wish to express thanks and appreciation to Catherine O'Leary, Lisa Barone, Linda Beverage, Kevin Craig, Ann M. Gannon, Ramon Melendez, Amy Mirand and Lucy Mirand, all of whom aided in various ways in the preparation of these volumes.

Finally, we wish to acknowledge the support of the National Cancer Institute, American Cancer Society, Pacific Northwest Regional Commission for their generous support of the 13th International Cancer Congress.

Edwin A. Mirand

Preface to Part A

All efforts to control cancer are defined and underscored by the unique coalescence of research, treatment, and educational activities, and are gauged by the impact these activities ultimately have on patient survival and quality of life. New and evolving information about cancer — generated both in and from laboratory and clinical settings — has virtually erased the vestigial "unidisciplinary" approach to the disease. Today's efforts to control cancer integrate extensive basic research, the vanguard of all clinical practice; treatment strategies and modalities that have been developed, tested, and implemented through multidisciplinary collaboration; and educational activities designed to promote professional and public awareness of the disease.

This volume of plenary lectures contains a plethora of cancer information, brought together under the aegis of disease management and cancer control. Topics deal with such timely issues and controversies as the recent trends in cancer treatment, the historical relevance of cancer epidemiology, the rationale for creating specific oncologic disciplines, and the role biology plays in the understanding of malignancy. Central to this volume is the emphasis on collaboration, both within and across institutions, disciplines, and nations.

Edwin A. Mirand

PLENARY CONGRESS LECTURES

The Role of National Efforts in Developing
Coordinated Programs on International Oncology.
*Murphy, G. P., Buffalo, NY USA.

The Role of Organization in Cancer Control.
*Wilcox, F. J., Eau Clarire, WI USA.

Why Surgical Oncology? Douglass, H. O.,
Buffalo, NY USA.

Advances in Cancer Therapeutics: Chemotherapy.
*De Vita, V. T., Jr., Bethesda, MD USA.

Cancer Epidemiology: Past, Present and
Future. *Muir, C. S., Lyon, France.

Recent Progress in Radiation Oncology.
*Tubiana, M., Paris, France.

The Role of Intensive Chemoradiotherapy and
Marrow Transplantation in the Treatment of
Disseminated Malignant Disease. *Thomas, E. D.,
Seattle, WA USA.

The Development and Clinical Application of
Hormone Receptor Concepts. *Jensen, E. V.,
Chicago, IL USA. (By Title Only)

Biology and Oncology: Regulation of Growth,
Differentiation and Malignancy. *Sachs, L.,
Rehovot, Israel.

Tumor Immunology Revisited. *Klein, G.,
Stokholm, Sweden. (By Title Only)

Environmental Mutagens, Carcinogens and Tumor
Promoters. *Sugimura, T., Tokyo, Japan.
(By Title Only)

**Please note: Papers that are listed as "By Title
Only" were presented at the 13th International
Cancer Congress, but are not included in these
volumes.**

13th International Cancer Congress, Part A
Current Perspectives in Cancer, pages 3–23
© 1983 Alan R. Liss, Inc., 150 Fifth Avenue, New York, NY 10011

THE ROLE OF NATIONAL EFFORTS IN DEVELOPING COORDINATED
PROGRAMS ON INTERNATIONAL ONCOLOGY

Gerald P. Murphy, M.D., D.Sc.

Institute Director
Roswell Park Memorial Institute
Buffalo, N.Y. 14263

The need to coordinate programs aimed at the cure and
control of cancer is undeniable. Disparities between potential and actual control of cancer can on occasion be disappointing. Ironically, eras of rapid advance in the number
and scope of activities relevant to cancer control actually
may experience initially a frustrating increase in these
disparities. Specialization of interest in cancer by affilia-
tion with a particular research discipline or service approach may sometimes lead to gaps, duplication, disjointed
efforts, or failure to pursue basic insights through to
clinical application. The coordination of cancer research
and service, therefore, is a critical consideration in the
development of effective efforts to control cancer.

The term "Renaissance man" confirms the existence and
the passing of an age when gifted individuals could be expected independently to remain conversant and effective in
all fields of knowledge. While it probably remains true that
individual creativity and initiative are the key ingredients
in the advance of scientific knowledge, it also consistently
is true that the most significant individual findings now
typically arise through the integration of several existing
disciplines or techniques. The nineteenth century development of research specialties shifted the locus of coordinated
efforts from the individual laboratory or clinic to the university medical school or research centers. Despite the
natural individual preference for independence and self-
sufficiency coupled with the widely voiced abhorrence of
bureaucracies necessitating external accountability, collaborative dependencies, committee meetings, etc., still the

observed abundance of voluntary associations and functional networks strikingly demonstrates an inherent impetus toward efforts to develop coordinated oncology programs.

The diversity in size, scope, and approach of specific associations reflects adaptation to local attributes and precedents, but the variety also reinforces the underlying observation that collaboration is universally inevitable when creative, effective individuals seek to achieve broader goals.

The turn of the twentieth century marked the transition from research with relevance for cancer to research targeted upon cancer, as exemplified in the establishment in 1898 of my own institution, Roswell Park Memorial Institute, as the first governmental support for a dedicated clinical cancer research unit. The early twentieth century also provided the first inter-institutional integration of researchers interested in cancer. That period saw the forerunners of the current major approaches to the coordination of research efforts, such as the following:

Forerunners of Current
Major Approaches to Coordination

PROFESSIONAL SOCIETIES:
  American Association for Cancer Research (1907)
  Japanese Pathological Society (1905)
JOURNALS:
  Revue des Maladies Cancereuses (1896)
  Zeitschrift fur Krebsforschung (1904)
  Bulletin du Cancer (1911)
  Journal of Cancer Research (1916)
  Gann (1907)
INTERNATIONAL CONGRESSES: Heidelberg (1906)
                          Madrid (1933)
PUBLIC VOLUNTARY AGENCIES:
  American Society for the Control of Cancer (1913)
  Japanese Association for Cancer Research (1915)

Today the complexities of research and new cancer control strategies may exceed the capabilities of individual local institutions or individuals. Scientific researchers must stay abreast of relevant reports which cross the traditional disciplines of biology, chemistry, physics, etc. Investigators involved in, for example, in vitro studies must achieve further development of their research leads through

collaboration with researchers involved in animal model systems and clinical trials. Clinical researchers must coordinate
a team which can incorporate into patient studies the diverse
contributions of surgery, chemotherapy, radiation therapy,
immunology, and supportive care. Reliance upon community
medical practitioners, with their particular knowledge of
the individual patient and the local setting, for delivery
of care requires a concerted effort to disseminate results
and promote application of the latest cancer knowledge. In
short, coordination is essential to enhance the cumulative
impact of individual cancer research and control activities.

INTERNATIONAL ONCOLOGY

Given then the need for coordinated cancer programs,
at what level should this integration occur? Certainly the
desire to cure and control cancer is worldwide, and many aspects of oncology are appropriately addressed at an international level. The credibility of the term "international
oncology" is evident in the responsibilities and services of
the International Union Against Cancer (UICC). In general,
these international responsibilities include:

1) fostering collaborative research
2) enhancing the training of personnel
3) coordinating services
4) disseminating information
5) assisting local and regional initiatives

Several references to specific UICC projects can illustrate
the realm of international oncology. The most immediately
apparent example is this International Cancer Congress,
which provides a worldwide forum to exchange ideas and com-
municate results on cancer research, therapy, control and
prevention.

The recently published UICC International Directory of
Specialized Cancer Research and Treatment Establishments
compiles a synopsis of the organization, resources, and activities of cancer centers throughout the world. The UICC Committee on International Collaborative Activities (CICA) also
has been instrumental in initiation of an International Cancer
Patient Data Exchange System, a patient registration network
facilitating information sharing between European and American
cancer centers. In collaboration with the National Cancer

Institute of the United States (NCI), an international computerized reference service, the International Cancer Research
Data Bank (ICRDB) has been maintained since 1974. The ICRDB
data base incorporates information on:

1) recently published literature (CANCERLIT)
2) current projects (CANCERPROJ)
3) current protocol studies (CANCERPROT)

and is accessible through the on-line capabilities of CANCER-
LINE. The system provides the basis for the Directory of
Cancer Research Information Resources and specialized reports
(<u>Cancergrams</u>) of abstracts of recently published articles in
a particular field which have appeared in the more than 3000
journals monitored.

In addition, International Scientist to Scientist Communication has represented a major UICC objective. The International Cancer Research Technology Transfer Program
(ICRETT) has provided to date over 600 awards since 1975 supporting researchers for travel, study and work at foreign
centers.

As in most collaborative endeavors, the variety of
activities to be integrated and the diverse skills of multi-
institutional agencies usually means that coordination will
not equate with absolute centralization of responsibilities.
In the field of international oncology, the UICC has shared
the role of integrating worldwide endeavors with the World
Health Organization (WHO) and the International Agency for
Cancer Research (IARC) in Lyon, France. These agencies and
their programs demonstrate the international scope of efforts
to promote the cure and control of cancer.

THE ROLE OF NATIONAL EFFORTS

While the term "international oncology" reflects the
fact that ultimately collaboration on cancer research and
service should be integrated at the international level, the
driving forces that stimulate and foster activities throughout the world must be closer and more responsive to the
local setting and its specific individuals and institutions.
One could draw an analogy with industry.

Each of the international cancer associations has en-

couraged the formation of regional groups that promote cooperation aimed at the priorities of specific sectors of the
world. The UICC has assisted the establishment of affiliations
such as:

Regional Associations of Cancer Institutes

- European Organization for Research on Treatment of Cancer
- Organization of European Cancer Institutes
- Scandinavian Cancer Union
- Latin American Association of Cancer Institutes
- Federation of Middle Eastern Cancer Organizations
- Asian Federation of Organizations for Cancer Research and
  Control
- COMECON

One of the older regional associations, EORTC, has evolved
into an extensive network of institutions in 13 countries
conducting nearly 100 clinical trials and publishes the
European Journal of Cancer & Clinical Oncology in collaboration with the European Association for Cancer Research.
Roswell Park is one of 10 U.S. centers joining 12 Latin
American centers in a Collaborative Cancer Treatment Program
of the Pan-American Health Organization and NCI, with studies
addressing hematological malignancies, osteosarcomas, and advanced breast, gastric, and head and neck tumors.

NCI-PAHO Collaborative Cancer
Treatment Research Program

Argentina:
  Grupo Argentino de Tratamiento (GATLA), Academia Nacional
  de Medicina
  Grupo Argentino de Tratamiento de los Tumores Solidos
  (GATTS), Universidad del Salvador
  Instituto "Angel H. Roffo"

Brazil:
  Fundacao A. C. Camargo
  Instituto Nacional de Cancer

Chile:
  Universidad Catolica de Chile
  Hospital Luis Calvo Mackenna

Colombia:
  Instituto Nacional de Cancerologia, Ministerio de Salud
  Publica

Costa Rica:
  Hospital de Ninos, "Dr. Carlos Saenz Herrera"
  Hospital San Juan de Dios

Mexico:
  Hospital de Oncologia, Instituto Mexicano de Seguridad
  Social

Peru:
  Instituto Nacional de Enfermedades Neoplasicas (INEN)

United States:
  Vincent T. Lombardi Can. Res. Ctr., Georgetown University,
  M.D. Anderson Hospital and Tumor Institute, Memorial
  Sloan-Kettering Cancer Center, University of Wisconsin,
  Roswell Park Memorial Institute, Baylor University Medical
  Center, New York University Medical Center, Comprehensive
  Cancer Center for Florida, University of Miami, University
  of Maryland Cancer Center, Yale University

Uruguay:
  Hospital de Clinicas "Dr. Manuel Quintela"

Venezuela:
  Instituto de Oncologia "Luis Razetti"

    This report focuses, however, on the essential role
that national organizations must play in stimulating and
coordinating contributions to international oncology. This
Seattle Congress devotes a substantial portion of its program to subject areas which rely heavily upon the support
and assistance of national organizations, particularly
voluntary or community leagues and societies. Examples of
these responsibilities include the funding of community-
wide cancer control programs, public education, school programs, use of the mass media, cancer prevention interventions, smoking cessation campaigns, screening, accessible
diagnostic and treatment services, rehabilitation and
continuing care.

    One should stress the relevance of national efforts to
develop coordinated programs on international oncology to

the developing nations. Approximately 2/3 of the world population resides in Africa, Asia and Latin America. These nations should anticipate that the control of communicable diseases, the projected increase in life expectancy, and the introduction of lifestyle changes, workplace exposures and environmental effluents associated with industrialization will raise dramatically the significance of cancer as a community public health concern.[1] It has been noted that the transition from a preponderance of infectious diseases to a preponderance of non-communicable diseases occurred in China and Singapore within a single generation. Unfortunately, few developing nations currently have either the total number of medical professionals needed or a sufficient cadre of committed community leaders to mount an effective national cancer campaign. The UICC, therefore, must remain committed to efforts that promote the establishment of cancer organizations at the national level in developing countries.

In the United States, the role of national organizations and reliance on their capabilities is well established, assumed, and perhaps often taken for granted. The National Cancer Act of 1971 represented a benchmark in the development of national efforts in the U.S. to control cancer. This Act required the Director of the National Cancer Institute (NCI) to involve broad representation in the effort to plan a coordinated cancer research program and to enhance oncology services through stimulation of research and promotion of the implementation of new developments. The continued prominence of the NCI, its Director, the National Cancer Advisory Board, and the President's Cancer Panel indicates the significance and the nature of the responsibilities for leadership, advocacy, and coordination at the national level. These centralized functions are complemented by organizational efforts in the Division of Resources, Centers and Community Activities to extend resources and programs across the country. The U.S. also can count on a wealth of voluntary national associations. Professional affiliations such as the American Association for Cancer Research and the American Society of Clinical Oncology address the issue of information exchange among researchers. Institutional collaboration is the fundamental focus of organizations such as the Association of American Cancer Institutes and the Association of Community Cancer Centers. The Commission on Cancer of the American College of Surgeons illustrates the attention given to the development of criteria for determining the quality of patient care and training. Finally, the record of the American Cancer

Society demonstrates, beyond any other U.S. association, the potential for achieving interventions at the local level through community-wide organization. The American Cancer Society deserves special recognition for its ability to make cancer research and control a priority of the community.

NATIONAL ROLES IN COORDINATING PROGRAMS

Three fundamental roles for national efforts are:

1) activities inherently requiring a national perspective
2) national strategies to stimulate local activities
3) coordination of local resources and activities

Responsibilities inherently necessitating a national perspective include public health legislation, definition of standards of care, national data bases, and provisions for specialized services and an overall infrastructure. With regard to public health laws, this aspect is particularly relevant to developing countries. The pattern of disease, including cancer, in developing countries reflects primarily the economic and technological conditions of the countryside and urban centers. Although hospitals generally represent approximately 80% of health expenditures in developing nations, medical practitioners in developing countries readily confirm the need to enact public health measures that address community conditions. Given the tendency to focus upon major health institutions such as hospitals, national efforts may be appropriate to encourage these institutions to take on community outreach programs, particularly in the training of medical practitioners to undertake extramural commitments in the community setting. These steps are essential to achievement of the goal, established at the World Health Organization's conference at Alma Ata in 1978 on primary health care in developing countries, which called for "health for all by the year 2000".[2]

NATIONAL STANDARDS OF CARE

With regard to national standards of care, these criteria may apply to either the facilities available in local communities or their utilization. A small country such as Papua & New Guinea can report a national cancer control program based upon agreement on treatment protocols. In larger countries, such as Iran and Ireland, comprehensive cancer centers in capital cities maintain national centers for pathological diagnosis. In West Germany, screening services coordinated by the Deutsches Krebsforschung Zentrum in Heidelberg are mandated by law. And in India, regional comprehensive cancer centers in Ahmedabad and Bangalore cite their operation of rural cancer diagnostic camps to screen for early disease. Developing nations need to consider to what extent they wish to define optimal, attainable standards for the provision of cancer services in the community.

Maintenance of a centralized data registry should be a fundamental national responsibility. In the absence of data registration, identification of epidemiological patterns of disease and follow-up of patient cases become impossible. Such data registration must be supra-regional to assure observation of rare tumors, comparison of etiological factors in different regions, and follow-up of referral patterns that encompass a large region. Countries that do not currently collect mortality statistics, which may represent nearly 90% of developing nations, must be encouraged to establish cause-of-death reporting for all diseases. In carefully selected areas, the development of hospital and population-based registries should be encouraged for reliable estimates of cancer incidence. While cross-sectional reports from different countries are useful, time-series data from a single country usually are more revealing of disease mechanisms and the efficacy of cancer control interventions. The full usage of a data repository can include:

Uses of National Data Repositories

1. patterns of incidence
2. mortality rates
3. targeting high risk populations
4. patterns of patient care and survival
5. distribution of cancer services
6. environmental factors

Such registry efforts are underway in Bombay, Bangkok, and Singapore; and in European countries such as Austria, Bulgaria, and Romania the comprehensive cancer centers can rely on national mandate of requirements for reporting cases.

MEDICAL SYSTEM: SPECIALIZED SERVICES AND REFERRAL NETWORKS

A national perspective is necessary to review the availability of specialized cancer resources and provide a network of arrangements to assure accessibility to these referral facilities. In smaller countries, single institutions may establish a central facility, such as radiation therapy, as a regional service, as exemplified by the National Oncology Institute of Panama, which maintains the only radiation therapy facility in the country and arranges for the referral of approximately 90% of all cancer patients.[3] Some countries, such as Colombia, have defined a National Cancer Plan, which in Colombia combines a commitment to central facilities at the Instituo Nacional de Cancerologia (Colombian National Cancer Institute) in Bogota with a plan or decentralized diagnostic capabilities at 8 regional cancer units and a network of over 1000 volunteers promoting cancer prevention interventions. Typically, many nations have developed a cancer center in the capital, collaborating with the Ministry of Public Health, to direct attention throughout the country to cancer control. Examples include the National Cancer Institute at Cairo University, the Instituto de Oncologia "Luis Razetti" (Luis Razetti Institute of Oncology) in Caracas, and the National Cancer Control Center of the Department of Health in Manilla.

In larger countries, the network of specialized services and related infrastructure is dependent upon district or regional centers. Our neighbor Canada provides an excellent illustration, where each of the provinces has a designated comprehensive cancer center, such as the Princess Margaret Hospital of the Ontario Cancer Institute, and some such centers have designated subregional networks, such as units of the Ontario Cancer Foundation in Kingston, London, Ottawa, Thunder Bay and Windsor. In summary, the first major forum for national efforts in developing coordinated programs in international oncology is the establishment of core resources requiring a national perspective, such as:

Efforts Requiring a National Perspective

- Public health laws
- National standards for care
- Data repositories
- Specialized referral centers
- Collaboration network

NATIONAL STIMULATION OF LOCAL INITIATIVES

Returning to the original outline, facilitation of local initiatives represents a second major role for national efforts. Areas in which national organizations can implement strategies to stimulate local activities include:

Strategies to Stimulate Local Activities

- definition of national priorities
- promotion of international exchanges
- wide dissemination of new findings
- facilitation of regional collaborations

Priorities need to be established at the national level in order to highlight the specific concerns of significance to the local community. This consideration is particularly relevant to developing countries which may have public health issues quite different from the general goals of international oncology as formulated by agencies representing technologically advanced societies. These priorities should take into account not only the patterns of disease in the country and the opportunities for prevention and control programs, but a national program can incorporate consideration of the unique service resources available in that community, and the implication of national traditions, social, economic, or political conditions. Once priorities are identified, cancer leagues and societies play a critical role in bringing these issues to the attention of the government and the national media. Acceptance of these goals by these national agencies can provide local activities with a baseline credibility and authorization which builds receptivity in the community setting.

INTERNATIONAL EXCHANGES

Visits between workers in different countries remain one of the most effective mechanisms for establishing an international exchange on oncology. Within developing countries, these exchanges can stimulate collaborative efforts in the definition of priorities and interventions particularly suited to developing nations. Exchanges between technologically advanced countries and developing nations can expedite the dissemination of new techniques and research approaches. These exchanges should not be limited to scientific centers, for national voluntary leagues and associations similarly can benefit through visits which highlight the roles of these societies in different settings.

The UICC has maintained three major travel fellowship programs, the Yamagiwa-Yoshida Memorial International Studies under the auspices of the Japan National Committee, the Fellowships of the Cancer Research Campaign, and the Eleanor Roosevelt International Cancer Fellowships supported by the American Cancer Society. Several nations have sponsored scholarship programs to benefit directly their country. La Asociacion Argentina del Cancer together with the Foundation Alfredo Fortabat offered four fellowships to attend this Seattle Congress. The Ligue Nationale Francaise Contre le Cancer has awarded international fellowships to bring recognized foreign researchers who are willing to introduce a new technique or idea into a French cancer research laboratory. In many cases, bilateral agreements have fostered such exchanges. The Soviet Union has established such arrangements with France, Italy, and the United States. The United States has been most active in bilateral agreements through the NCI since 1972. U.S. bilateral agreements currently involve:

U.S. Bilateral Agreements

- USSR Agreement for Cooperation in the Fields of Medical Science and Public Health
- Japanese Society for the Promotion of Science
- Polish People's Republic Agreement
- French Institute National de la Sante et de la Recherche Medicale
- Arab Republic of Egypt
- Ministry of Science and Technology of the Federal Republic of Germany
- People's Republic of China Accord for Cooperation in Science & Technology
- National Cancer Institute of Milan
- National Institute of Oncology (Hungarian People's Republic)

National agencies play a key role in these exchanges, which promote the coordination of international oncology.

National cancer congresses also have a valuable role to play in stimulating local cancer initiatives. For example, the Fourth Cancer Congress of Colombia, jointly sponsored by the Colombian National Cancer Institute, the Colombian

League for the Control of Cancer, the Colombian Cancer
Society and the Colombian Society of Radiotherapy, combined
such valuable and diverse elements as a national congress,
a major symposium on cancer research, refresher courses on
cancer services, and seminars on education of the community
in cancer control.[4] Similar national meetings are hosted by
cancer societies of Japan, Argentina and the Phillipines.
Dissemination of information, then, on the current status
of cancer research and services should be a commitment of
a national organization in developing countries.

The development of regional cancer centers should be
encouraged at the national level. Comprehensive cancer
centers at the regional level can stimulate interaction between bench scientists and practicing clinicians, foster
multidisciplinary care, and serve as local points for dissemination of new developments in the field. Cancer centers
should be selected on the basis of the excellence of their
expertise and the role they can play for a given geographic
region. In some countries, associations are dedicated to
fostering the collaboration of cancer centers. These
associations include:

National Associations of Cancer Centers

- French Federation of Anticancer Centers
- Association of Italian Cancer Institutes
- Scientific Council for Multidisciplinary Study of
  Malignant Neoplasms (USSR Academy of Medical Sciences)
- Swiss Working Group on Clinical Cancer Research (SAKK)
- Turkish Federation of Oncology Centers
- Association of American Cancer Institutes (AACI)

Such centers need not be constrained by walls or institutional affiliations. At the level of particular research
disciplines, scientific academies, professional societies,
and those concerned with the publication of scientific and
technical journals can provide a valuable resource through
organization at the national level.

The second major reason for developing coordinated programs in international oncology at the national level, then,
is that organizations within developing countries can bring
together incentives for local cancer control initiatives.
Programs such as the definition of national priorities, promotion of international exchanges, forums for dissemination

of findings, and encouragement of associations of centers and professionals can play a key role in stimulating cancer research and control endeavors throughout the country.

One should also stress the role of national efforts to assist in the coordination of local resources and activities. A comprehensive cancer control program should integrate:

Elements of Comprehensive Cancer Control Programs

- Education
- Environmental Monitoring
- Epidemiological data
- Screening and early diagnosis
- Interdisciplinary care
- Rehabilitation services and continuing care
- Community support
- Research

Few local institutions can direct such a wide array of interventions without the support and assistance of regional and national organizations. With regard to education, many local institutions will need aid in the recruitment of medical and non-medical volunteers for projects to educate the general public on prevention and early detection of cancer. A major problem of many cancer leagues and societies is the difficulty experienced in getting health professionals to commit to roles in non-scientific activities of these organizations. Five Scandinavian cancer associations recently sponsored a Scandinavian Workshop on Doctor Involvement to identify means to involve general and community physicians in educating the public about cancer.[5] Cancer societies were cited as key agents in securing the cooperation of groups such as health personnel and schoolteachers. The first step should be advocacy of national policies on undergraduate medical training that would emphasize coverage in the curricula of aspects such as prevention, screening, primary care, and psychological support for cancer patients. In many developing countries, however, perhaps only 10% of the rural population is served by physicians. In countries with a shortage of doctors, cancer societies must identify community health workers or nurses who can be utilized in public education, and regional workshops may be necessary to train relevant manpower. Some aids are available for the task. For example, a special UICC project produced a Manual on Cancer Education in Schools, which has been presented at regional implementation conferences.

The variation in frequency of different types of cancer
means that cancer leagues and societies should identify
public education interventions aimed at the types of cancer
most prevalent in their own country. Certainly the concern
for exposure to cigarette smoke, the sun, and vinyl chlorides
should be widespread, and one should emphasize particularly
the importance of national anti-smoking campaigns. These
campaigns are not futile, as evidenced by the sharp decrease
in the number of smokers in the informed population of health
professionals in Australia, Scandinavian countries, the United
Kingdom, and the U.S.[6] The Third European Symposium on
Smoking Control held in Budapest in 1981 emphasized that patterns of tobacco consumption vary considerably from one
nation to another, and thus an effort at the national level
is imperative. In any public education campaign, a national
society can play a key role in the development of audiovisual
materials. The UICC must maintain its commitment to providing
for developing countries publications, audiovisual materials,
and expertise references in English, French, Spanish and
Portuguese which can be adapted further for other nationali-
ties.

The need for national assistance to regional data repositories has been indicated previously. While hospital and
local registries are important for achievement of complete
cancer reporting, and can be targetted to data relevant to
local studies of interest, coordination at the supra-regional
level is necessary to assure sufficient coverage of rare
tumors, comparison of regional patterns of exposures and
disease, and follow-up of treatment and survival results in
a referral network.

Cancer leagues and societies have a major role to play
directly, or in aiding local institutions, in the promotion
of cancer screening and early detection programs.[7] These
efforts are relevant particularly to sites of disease such
as cervix, breast, lung, and colon/rectum. Many comprehensive cancer centers have established early detection clinics
for assymptomatic patients, such as the unit at the Louvain
Cancer Center in Belgium which screens 15,000 clients annually. An interesting collaborative effort is underway in
Peru.[8] Cervical screening is compulsory for all hospitals
and health centers in Lima, and the slides are collected,
processed and followed-up free of charge through a central

service of the Instituto Nacional de Enfermedades Neoplasicas
(Peruvian National Neoplastic Disease Institute), which also
trains 10 cytotechnics annually. In Arequipa, The Goyeneche
Hospital Tumor Unit reaches throughout the community through
detection subcenters in Arequipa, Puno and Mollendo. At the
national level, associations can define projects aimed at
concerns particular to that community.

NATIONAL COLLABORATIVE TREATMENT GROUPS

For identified cancer cases, collaborative treatment
groups can contribute a valuable resource in defining appropriate multidisciplinary care and follow-up. The importance of study design and evaluation to the advance of
knowledge concerning the clinical management of cancer can
not be overstated. The typical multicenter cooperative group
will involve designated participating centers, a centralized
data collection unit, specialty units such as pathology confirmation, a steering committee of the participants, and an
advisory group of outside expertise for evaluation of trials.
In the United States, the NCI has assisted the formation of
over 17 cooperative groups. The National Cancer Institute of
Canada (NCIC) has a Clinical Trials Group conducting studies
in 1982 in such diverse areas as melanoma, ovarian cancer,
pediatric tumors, osteogenic sarcoma, and hematologic
malignancies. The U.K. Cancer Trials Register, operating
under the aegis of the Coordinating Committee on Cancer
Research, the British Association of Surgical Oncology, and
the Medical Research Council's Head Office, centralizes up-
to-date information on current Phase III trials in order
to reduce the number of small, unproductive studies and
to reduce unnecessary duplication of related trial protocols.[9]
Collaborative treatment groups are equally relevant to
small countries mounting a program based on a number of
individual hospitals.

Some leagues and societies have devoted much energy and
resources to the promotion of facilities for the rehabilitation and continuing care of patients with advanced cancer.
In Peru, the Liga Peruana de Lucha Contra el Cancer pro-
motes CAPANINEN, a support group dedicated to children
with cancer and their parents. And some associations have
recognized the services needed to aid terminal cancer patients, responding with commitments such as the Sri Lanka
Cancer Society's terminal home and rehabilitation project,

and the many other hospice programs in operation throughout the world.

National cancer organizations can provide the focal point for bringing together the diverse sectors of the community with interests related to cancer. One is struck by the history of the Swedish Cancer Society, which was founded in 1951 as a joint venture of:

Founding Members of
Swedish Cancer Society

- Political parties
- Confederation of Trade Unions
- Swedish Employer's Confederation
- Swedish Broadcasting Corp.
- National Union of Journalists
- Professional Medical Associations
- Federation of Swedish County Councils

This coalition dramatically demonstrates the catalytic impact of unifying such diverse, influential community representatives into a single organization to provide community support for cancer patient care and cancer control endeavors.

FUND RAISING

One should stress the need for national efforts to raise funding for cancer research. We must recognize that the private sector, great as its commitment to research and development may be, cannot adequately finance the necessary level of biomedical research desired. Although many cancers can be controlled and will be controlled in our lifetime through application of current knowledge, the key contributions to the long-term advance of medicine, enhancement of oncology services, and improvement of community health care will come from the clinical and pre-clinical research insights under development in pilot studies or still at the conceptual stage.

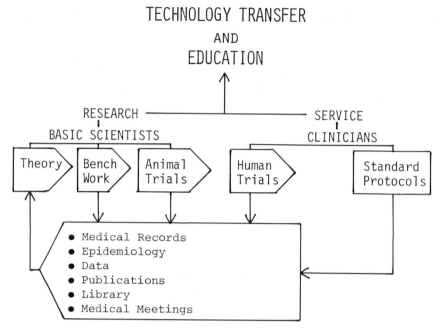

TECHNOLOGY TRANSFER
AND
EDUCATION

Guidelines for Developing a Comprehensive Cancer Centre
UICC Technical Report Series - Volume 53

A primary responsibility of cancer leagues and societies, therefore, must be to raise money for cancer research. Third world nations can benefit to a limited degree from the experience of successful voluntary associations. The Danish Cancer Society is funded in part by the national lottery. The Swedish Cancer Society has the support of the King Gustaf V. Jubilee Fund. The National Cancer Institute of Canada has awarded grants and fellowships since 1947. These resources are examples of an essential function which is necessary to support the advances in technological capabilities, the increasing research specialization, and the pace at which research insights are developing.

In summary, national efforts are vital to the coordination of the diverse elements necessary to a comprehensive cancer control program. Voluntary societies and agencies, in particular, have a role to play in such areas as:

Elements of a Comprehensive Cancer Control Program

- Education
- Environmental monitoring
- Data exchange
- Screening and early detection
- Confirmation of diagnosis
- Treatment collaboration
- Rehabilitation
- Community support
- Research

Oncology truly is an international field. One should apologize to those associations or organizations who have not been mentioned in this brief report who are conducting exemplary work in response to some of the responsibilities we have defined for national efforts. All are encouraged to review the International **Directory** of Specialized Cancer Research and Treatment Establishments, which provides a wealth of references to active and effective projects in diverse settings.

This report has stressed the responsibilities that national organizations should face up to in order to further the development of coordinated programs in international oncology. To conclude these remarks, it is important to stress that international associations, such as the UICC, must make a further commitment to assist developing countries in undertaking these roles. The genesis for this speech came from a presentation by Dr. A.O. Williams of Nigeria at a May 29, 1981 UICC Advisory Meeting on the potential role of the UICC Programme on Cancer Campaign and Organization in third world countries. He defined 10 UICC projects which could facilitate these national efforts, and cited these aids:

1) to establish close contacts with local, indigenous organizations in developing countries.
2) to contact appropriate **Health** authorities in developing countries without national associations with a view to stimulating their formation.
3) to arrange consultative visits between established national organizations and groups in **developing** nations.
4) to collaborate with other international and regional agencies in these endeavors.

5) to stress the development of materials and audio-visual aids relevant to programs of developing nations.
6) to bring the discussion of national organizations to the agenda of international meetings and congresses.
7) to encourage studies directed at the particular needs of developing countries.
8) to raise funding support specifically for the development of national programs in developing countries.
9) to organize within the UICC to give attention to priorities and policies regarding developing countries and to assist in follow-up and implementation.
10) to promote throughout the world an awareness of the significance of cancer control to the health of communities in developing nations.

This agenda represents a major undertaking. I have no doubt of the need for the effort and its merit. National organizations will play the key role in developing and coordinating the field of oncology on an international scope. With your assistance, an effective program can, will, and has been mounted.

References

A.O. Williams, The Potential Role of the UICC Programme on Cancer Campaign and Organization in Third World Countries. Presented at UICC Advisory Meeting. Geneva. May 29, 1981.

Journal of the American Medical Association. Medical News. Vol. 247. No. 10. March 12, 1982. p. 1383.

Committee on International Collaborative Activities (CICA) (1978). International Directory of Specialized Cancer Research and Treatment Establishments. UICC Technical Report Series-Volume 33. Geneva. p. 330.

UICC Information (1981). Union Internationale Contre Le Cancer. Geneva. No. 5. Nov-Dec., p.3.

Ibid., p. 4.

Third European Symposium on Smoking Control, Budapest. October 1981.

Union Internationale Contra Le Cancer. UICC Information. Geneva. No. 5. Nov-Dec. 1981. p. 2.

Committee on International Collaborative Activities (CICA). International Directory of Specialized Cancer Research and Treatment Establishments. UICC Technical Report Series. Volume 33. Geneva. 1978. p. 335.

A.R. Currie. Letter to the Editor. British Journal of Cancer. 1982. 45. p. 648.

13th International Cancer Congress, Part A
Current Perspectives in Cancer, pages 25–29
© 1983 Alan R. Liss, Inc., 150 Fifth Avenue, New York, NY 10011

THE ROLE OF ORGANIZATION IN CANCER CONTROL

Francis J. Wilcox

Honorary Life Member, Board of Directors,
American Cancer Society, 131 South Barstow Street,
Eau Claire, WI 54701

To discuss the role of organization in the fight against cancer requires that we look at what has developed in the past and what organizations are doing today and we must understand what is meant by an organization before we can make any effort for planning for the future. The organization we are referring to is a group of people who have brought themselves together as a broad-based part of the community, including doctors, lawyers, ordinary people, professionals, teachers, governmental workers, the entire broad spectrum of community people; and organized for the purpose of carrying on the most efficient and effective campaign against cancer possible. Traditionally, the role of the non-medical organization was centered around patient care motivated by their love of fellow man, the churches and the charitable organizations of the older day built, maintained and staffed hospitals, nursing homes and places for medical care. They did this because there was no other agency to do so, and they filled the void of necessity and did a magnificent job.

Early in the history of cancer treatment, the oncologists concentrated their efforts on research and the improvement of therapy for a better chance of survival and the International Union Against Cancer followed that pattern. Its early programs were centered around scientific research, the development of improved protocols of surgical treatment and other therapeutic methods. The organizations throughout the world which joined the Union followed the traditional pattern of concern for the creation and support of facilities for the care and treatment of cancer patients, hospitals, nursing homes and detection centers. Gradually, the

scientific community developed more and better realization
of the cancer cell itself, how it developed and how it grew
and of the importance of early detection and of the importance of team treatments and care of the cancer patient and
his family. With that realization, the government and
medical community gradually began to assume the role of
creating, supporting and maintaining the necessary facilities which were beyond the power of non-governmental
organziations to create and to support.

During the early days of the Congresses, little or no
reference was made to the non-medical organizations who
were members of the Union. However, commencing with Tokyo
in 1966, the first committee on organization was created,
and from there on under the leadership of Dr. Denoix, Dr.
Taylor and Mildred Allen, the International Union became
more and more interested in the work and the importance of
cancer organizations. Through the creation in Houston in
1970 of the Commission on Organization, then at Florence,
Italy in 1974 of the program of organization, the organizational members of the Union were given a direct voice on
its council and executive committee. Now we find the
non-medical organizations are a dynamic and leading force
in promoting the health of the public. They mean more
service and participation by more and more people who
inform themselves and help solve problems. They concentrate
in the direct support of research through fund-raising and
through encouraging and persuading governments to increase
their support of research. They work in the field of
professional education by providing funds for scholarships
and for seminars for the persons in the health field.
Also, they can be effective in funding and persuading
medical schools to establish chairs of oncology and to
increase the amount of oncological training for doctors.
Another field has been the shortening of the time from
laboratory discovery to clinical application through the
support and training of specialists and the conducting of
educational programs for the practitioner. The organizations
themselves have a particularly effective role of fact-finders
and interpreter of facts, they assist in gathering such
information as to the size of groups and the effects of
various programs and in the awareness of the public as to
the nature of cancer, the curability and treatment of
cancer and how they can best protect themselves. The study
conducted by the New Zealand Cancer Society indicated that
the most effective tool in promoting self-examination of
breasts and early screening for breast cancer was the work

of the organization in distributing pamphlets and in leading discussions with women's groups in direct contact. This was again confirmed by the findings of the Italian group with respect to cervical cancer who found that to get satisfactory results an essential condition for early screening was personal invitation and conduct by individuals of organizational societies. Finally the organizations have and now are carrying on a wide program of service and care for the cancer patient, not of the traditional nature of institutional care, but in the promotional programs of rehabilitation and in working with the cancer patient and his family in meeting the shock of cancer and providing personal service, giving transportation and in home care, and in the more recent field of prevention in working with the public to make them aware of what they can do to reduce their chances of obtaining cancer. Perhaps the best example of the effectiveness of organization in rehabilitation is the developpment of the Reach for Recovery Program in continental Europe through the work of Mrs. Timothy. Another in the field of patient and family care is the development of the role of the hospices by Cecily Saunders of England and the home-care concept which has been spread throughout many parts of the world by the organizational members of the Union.

What is the future role of the non-medical organization in the fight against cancer? It would appear that a free and independent and undirected research program can best be created and supported by the availability of funds that are not channelled through governmental institutions. The necessity of budget restraints and cost-effective tests that are a part of governmental support can be cut short by private funding. An alternate source of funding gives competition in the applications for research and sharpens the interest of the researcher and makes the chances of the most effective research being funded improved. A typical example of a massive form of research that could not have been funded by any government was the investment of over $9,000,000 by the American Cancer Society in the clinical research with the use of Interferon, and in epidemiological research the massive cancer prevention study of over a million people which is being repeated this year for another 5-year period in order to obtain basic knowledge on the effect of lifestyles. This type of research could not be carried on without the presence of an effective organization of the type we are discussing. It would be a step backward if the sole source of research money was channelled through bureaucratic sources of government even though they may be the largest single source. The interest of the rehabilitation of the cancer patient, of the improvement of the quality of life of the cancer patient after his treatment and of the support for the patient and his family in the psychological impact of cancer is a peculiarly appropriate field for the organizations to concern themselves with. People who care, informed people who understand and realize the problem, can be mobilized through such an organization to deal with the local problems on the local level with less cost and more effectiveness and more sense of love and support than any other organization. The type of national organization that has been carried on in Finland to support the cancer patients through local facilities, clubs and visitation and meeting places, is an example of what can be accomplished through the organization of dedicated people in this field.

In the field of prevention, dealing with the lifestyle of people which the scientific community tells us with greater and greater emphasis may be the eventual way in which cancer will be controlled or reduced. There is a tremendously important role for the organization to carry out. Informed neighbor who gives an example and a motivation for lifestyle changes is the only effective method. Governmental prohibitions have never been successful. The role of government in prevention is the control of identified carcinogen hazards and the regulation of their appearance in the marketplace and the role of the organization in identifying such hazards and in pressuring government to take appropriate steps can be extremely effective in many areas. It has also been found that the motivation necessary to have the public take the necessary steps for early detection can best be generated by the person-to-person contacts which a local organization can make, that publicity and media coverage and governmental edict do not have the same impact and will not produce the same percentage of results among the public at large, and so therefore in all 4 fields of research, education, patient care, prevention and early detection, the organization can and should in the future play an increasingly important role. In this era of financial restrictions and government cutbacks, the role of the organization must be evermore important and more prominent.

The thousands of dedicated people who have and are giving of themselves to the work of organizations of this Union are a force for the good of mankind; they daily prove their concern and love for their neighbor and their country. Untold numbers of people have been comforted and lives have been saved by their efforts. As we move more and more into the fields of prevention, management and concern and support for the cancer patient and his family, there will be an ever-increasing need for such organizations. May the Union and its members continue to foster and support their growth and efforts so that evermore lives may be saved.

13th International Cancer Congress, Part A
Current Perspectives in Cancer, pages 31–45
© 1983 Alan R. Liss, Inc., 150 Fifth Avenue, New York, NY 10011

WHY SURGICAL ONCOLOGY?

Harold O. Douglass, Jr., M.D.

Roswell Park Memorial Institute
666 Elm Street
Buffalo, New York 14263

In each major discipline of medicine, there has been a tendency for physicians treating cancer patients to separate into subspecialty groups. Thus, the discovery of the cytodestructive potential of radiation led to the separation of radiation oncologists from diagnostic radiology, first as a subspecialty and then as an independent medical discipline. Recognition of the antineoplastic potential of the mustard drugs, led a small group of physicians to search for other agents that might be effective in treating cancer, and the discovery of antimetabolites, alkylating agents, antibiotics and other agents. As the initial responses were seen mostly in hematologic malignancies, medical oncology developed as a hematology subspecialty, not becoming an independent specialty until the early 1970's.

In contrast, the surgical removal of malignant tumors is the oldest form of therapy and is still the chief form of curative treatment for most forms of cancer. Indeed, the first successful gastrectomy was performed by Billroth for a cancer of the antrum of the stomach. Improvements in anesthesia, the ready availability of blood and blood products, and the development of effective antibiotics prompted increasingly aggressive surgical procedures to remove not only the primary tumor site but also areas of regional spread. Breast amputations progressed to radical mastectomies and then to extended and super-radical

Supported in part by Gastrointestinal Tumor Study Group Grant CA 34184 and Eastern Cooperative Oncology Group Grant CA 12296.

mastectomies. The ultimate ablative procedure was the hemicorporectomy. However, it became apparent that increasingly more extensive resection rarely increased the potential for patient cure, while disfigurement and disability did increase. Thus, for many years there was little improvement on the results of abdominoperineal resection following the original work of Miles, and the super-radical mastectomy failed to increase survival over that which resulted from the Willy-Meyer/Halsted radical mastectomy as much as it increased the operative mortality and morbidity. In contrast to the approaches of the cancer surgeon, many surgical oncologists have taken different courses in treatment planning.

THE CANCER SURGEON AND THE SURGICAL ONCOLOGIST ARE NOT NECESSARILY THE SAME PERSON

The surgery of cancer has not been recognized as a separate surgical specialty because cancer plays such an important role in general surgical training. Thus surgeons ask, "What is different about surgical oncology?" or "What can the surgical oncologist do that I can't do?". Indeed, one university surgical chief, after hiring a surgical oncologist to participate in his training program, was heard to express the feeling, "I don't know what surgical oncology is, but now we have one". For surgeons, and non-surgeons alike, this short presentation may answer the question, "Why surgical oncology?".

While cancer surgeons were increasing the extent of ablative procedures, referring patients occasionally to radiation therapists or chemotherapists when it appeared that the surgical excision was incomplete, surgical oncologists were undertaking organized programs of patient evaluation, integrating the surgical procedure into a pre-planned multimodality therapeutic approach, developing planned follow-up procedures for the early detection of recurrence, and for the management of potential therapeutic complications. The surgical oncologist was developing a detailed knowledge of malignant disease, orienting a total patient care program towards the peculiarities of the natural history of each individual variety of cancer. He relied more heavily on the pathologist, asking to have the extent of primary disease in the resected specimen described in more detail, requesting more detailed knowledge of the number and site of involved and uninvolved lymph nodes, so that staging schema would permit the results of one therapeutic trial to be compared to those of another. Surgical oncology began to develop planned approaches to recurrent and metastatic disease, based on knowledge of the underlying pathophysiology. Integrated programs to enhance the survival of patients undergoing palliative surgery began to be developed, and resulted in the probable cure of a few patients.

The development of programs for cancer patient management in which surgery is just one of several therapeutic tools separates the surgical oncologist from the cancer surgeon. A few examples of these concepts, and their results, are presented as illustrative cases.

ADJUVANT AND MULTIMODAL TREATMENT TRIALS

For years, surgeons have told families (and perhaps themselves) that "we got it all out". Yet cure rates of 8-15 percent following resection for gastric cancer, for example, stand as mute testimony that they did not. There was little uniformity of opinion as to what constituted a "curative" operation, and even less conformity between the type of operation that should be performed and the extent of the resection actually done. There was just no way of resolving the discrepancies between a surgeon's operative note of a left hemicolectomy resecting from the right transverse colon and a pathology report that began "Specimen received consists of an 11 cm piece of colon with a circumferential tumor 2 cm from the distal end".

In 1973, a group of surgical oncologists in the Gastrointestinal Tumor Study Group (GITSG) sat down to define a curative gastric resection in terms to which all could agree (GITSG, 1982). The criteria established were far less rigid than those of the Japanese Research Society for the Study of Gastric Cancer. A curative gastrectomy was defined as one in which all known tumor was resected in an en-bloc procedure. A specimen could be divided only for technical reasons (such as to provide better exposure for a celiac axis lymph node dissection) and no discontiguous resections would be allowed. Peritoneal involvement could only be present at the site of the primary tumor. Removal of a tumor deposit separated from

SURVIVAL FOLLOWING CURATIVE RESECTION
FOR GASTRIC CANCER

Patient Group	Percent Alive at 2 Years		Percent Alive at 5 Years	
	Control	FU-MeCCNU	Control	FU-MeCCNU
All Patients	56%	68%	32%	46%
Stage II	72%	84%	48%	76%
Stage III	42%	60%	24%	30%
Distal Subtotal Resection	68%	78%	46%	62%
Proximal/Total Resection	34%	56%	12%	18%

Table 1. Controlled Adjuvant Trial of 5FU-MeCCNU Following Curative Resection for Gastric Cancer by the Gastrointestinal Tumor Study Group (GI 8174). Preliminary Results with Median Time On-Study at Four Years

the primary site (such as a distant lymph node or a peritoneal implant on an ovary) was encouraged, but even if this was the only site of known distant metastasis, the procedure could not be considered a curative resection. When the main tumor mass was adherent to an adjacent organ such as the pancreas, liver or mesocolon, it could not be "peeled off" that tissue. Rather, a portion of the adjacent organ had to be resected, even when resection mandated a partial colectomy, distal pancreatectomy or wedge resection of the liver. These combined resections were to be done as en-bloc procedures in order to fit the criteria of "curative".

Once the criteria of a curative resection were met, patients could be randomized either to receive chemotherapy or to be closely followed as a control group. Subsequently, two other similar cooperative group studies were initiated, but only the GITSG enforced the criteria of a "curative" resection.

Now, more than two years since the last patient entered the GITSG study, with more than half of the patients entered more than five years ago, preliminary results of this study have become available. This study suggests that the patients with the most advanced disease (with serosal invasion or lymph node metastases) and those with tumors that required either proximal or total gastrectomy for "curative" resection, were most likely to benefit from adjuvant chemotherapy. Two studies in other cooperative groups do not, as yet, confirm this advantage for adjuvant chemotherapy. Even in the control group, survival was markedly prolonged when criteria for curative resection were met (Table 1).

Many surgeons in the United States have long felt that gastric cancer in Japan was different from that seen elsewhere because of the high rate of long-term survivals (five-year cures occurring in more than half of patients in whom gastric cancer is diagnosed). While Stage I cancer is almost uniformly curable by surgery alone, the results reported by Japanese surgeons in Stage II and Stage III cancer seemed remarkably different (Table 2) with five-year survival rates of 50-60 percent, while reports from the United States and elsewhere noted five-year survival following resection for gastric cancer did not exceed 20 percent. In the GITSG study, the five-year survival of patients with Stage II gastric cancer who did not receive

RELATIVE SURVIVAL RATE OF GASTRIC CANCER IN
CONTROLLED TRIALS OF CHEMOTHERAPY AS
AN ADJUVANT TO SURGERY, FROM JAPAN

Trial	Stage	5-Year Survival of Controls	5-Year Survival with Chemotherapy
I	All	27%	25%
	II	44%	35%
	III	21%	20%
III	All	46%	47%
	II	49%	54%
	III	30%	21%
IV	All	65%	66%
	II	63%	66%
	III	52%	42%

Table 2. Controlled Trials of Adjuvant Chemotherapy in Japan.
Overall Improved Survival ("All" stages) Indicative
of the Increased Proportion of Early Cases Treated in
the Later Series. Improvement in Survival by Stage
in Controls (Stage II from 35 to 66%, Stage III from
20 to 42%) May Reflect the Acceptance of Surgeons of
the Standardized More Radical Resections Recommended
by the Japanese Research Society (Japanese Research
Society for Gastric Cancer, 1981).

adjuvant chemotherapy is estimated to approximate 50 percent while that of patients with Stage III gastric cancer is more than 20 percent. For patients who received adjuvant chemotherapy, five-year survival rates for patients with Stage II and Stage III gastric cancer are estimated at 75 and 45 percent, respectively. While these results do not duplicate the Japanese experience, they more closely approximate the reports from Japan than they do the earlier reports (might one call them historical controls?) from the United States.

A somewhat different type of integration of surgical therapy into multimodal treatment is reflected in the "modern" management of osteosarcoma. Since this is a malignancy of the teenage years, the criteria of five-year survival are not appropriate. Instead, we should consider 50-year survival as the objective of treatment. Despite the relative rarity of this tumor, a number of fairly complex multimodal therapeutic programs have been introduced in an attempt to reverse the historical tumor mortality rate of 80 to 90 percent. Most of the more successful osteosarcoma protocols now insert chemotherapy as the initial treatment, administered either systemically as combinations of drugs or locally by intra-arterial infusion. The timing of surgical ablation is then scheduled into the chemotherapy program, which then continues following tumor removal.

The results of these combined approaches (with 50 percent or more of patients expected to survive more than five years (Douglass, 1978) encouraged the surgical oncologist to more closely examine his operative procedure in an attempt to improve patient rehabilitation. Since osteosarcoma most commonly occurs in the region of the knee, the initial emphasis was to salvage femoral length by transmedullary amputation, for a more functional prosthesis, fitted in the operating room, and permitting the teenager to leave the hospital already walking on a prosthesis. Resections in the pelvis and of the humerus were also successfully performed, salvaging the limb, as the surgical oncologist began to recognize that the critical surgical margin was not the two or three feet between the tumor and the fingers or toes, but rather the few centimeters between the tumor and the proximal line of resection. These concepts have led to a search for a bone substitute and an attempt to salvage the extremity. Even a deformed or

SURVIVAL FOLLOWING RESECTION FOR OSTEOSARCOMA

Investigator or Group	Program	Survival
CALGB	Adriamycin	50% disease-free at 24 months
SWOG	Compadri I	55% disease-free at 36 months
	Compadri II	73% alive at 12 months
Jaffe	VCR-HDM-LV	58% disease-free at 18 months
Rosen	VCR-HDM-LV-Adr	68% disease-free at 24 months
RPMI	Adr-DDP	64% disease-free at 36 months

Table 3. Results of Uncontrolled Adjuvant Chemotherapy Trials in Osteosarcoma.

shortened extremity is vastly superior to our current best prosthetic capability. Two types of bone substitutes have had a fairly large trial: specially fabricated metallic devices such as the vitalium distal femur and knee and the cryopreserved bone allographs. Neither is the perfect replacement: morbidity remains significant. However, in the 1980's there are a number of long-term survivors with retained extremities, whereas only a decade ago there were few survivors, all of whom had been treated by radical amputations (Table 3).

Perhaps the ultimate integration of surgery into multimodality therapy is in the new trials for the management of patients with small cell lung cancer, in which patients with localized small cell lung cancer initially receive chemotherapy and are radiated. If, following treatment, the tumor is still found to be localized, pulmonary resection is performed (Broder, 1977). Thus, there has been a reversal of roles. Rather than surgical excision followed by radiation or chemotherapy to "mop up residual tumor, chemotherapy and radiation are the main therapeutic thrusts, the role of surgery being relagated to the removal of residual gross tumor (here surgery is the "adjuvant" therapy).

SURGICAL APPROACHES TO RECURRENT AND
METASTATIC DISEASE

Selected patients with metastases to the liver or lung, with little or no metastatic disease elsewhere, can be candidates for a direct surgical approach to these tumors. Since the median survival of patients with liver metastases ranges between four and eight months, dependant on the source of tumor metastases and the extent of metastatic involvement of the liver, patients with solitary or a few localized metastases from cancers of the colon and rectum, from melanomas, soft tissue tumors, gastric and pancreatic tumors and from other primary sites may be best managed by a direct approach: resection, hepatic artery ligation or infusion chemotherapy. In 1977, as a result of a nation wide survey, Foster showed that the five-year survival rate following the resection of liver metastases approached 20 percent (Foster, 1978). A Mayo Clinic study reported that 15 of 36 patients with solitary liver metastases were alive five years later, although six subsequently died of recurrent cancer (Adson 1980). However, no patients with multiple

metastases survived five years. At Roswell Park Memorial
Institute, we found the median survival of patients
following resection of solitary metastases of colorectal
cancers to approach 48 months with more than 30 percent
alive after five years.

The solitary metastasis is an uncommon lesion but the
surgical oncologist will search for these patients since
their potential to benefit from resection is so great.
When patients are found to have multiple or unresectable
liver metastases, alternative therapies, including hepatic
artery ligation and intra-arterial infusion chemotherapy,
can be offered. The therapeutic advantage of hepatic
arterial therapy lies in the fact that all but the periphery
of a metastatic nodule relies on the hepatic artery for its
oxygen and nutrient supply, whereas the hepatic parenchyma
receives half of its oxygen needs and 90 percent of its
nutrients from the portal vein. Thus, ligation of the
hepatic artery is usually well tolerated in absence of liver
decompensation or jaundice and when the portal vein is
patent. Extensive central necrosis of the metastatic
deposits (sometimes resulting in abscess formation within
the necrotic tumor mass) is the frequent result of the
metastatic dependency on the hepatic artery in-flow. It
has been our experience in patients with angiographically
demonstrated vascular tumors (e.g., carcinoids, sarcomas
and islet cell tumors) often regress most markedly after
hepatic artery ligation (Berjian, 1980). However, patients
whose metastases are not hypervascular, such as those with
metastatic colorectal cancer, can benefit from this
procedure. At Roswell Park Memorial Institute, a case-
matching study (matching age, sex, tumor site, differentiation
and extent of metastases in liver) showed that patients
treated by hepatic artery ligation survived a median of 55
weeks, twice that of the controls (median survival 28 weeks -
up-dated from Evans, 1979).

Long-term infusion chemotherapy via a surgically placed
hepatic artery catheter has several advantages over
treatment via transfemorally placed catheters due to the
reduction in gastrointestinal bleeding and ulceration that
follows ligation of the right gastric and gastroduodenal
arteries as well as other collaterals supplying the stomach
and duodenum (which are infused by the high concentration
of chemotherapeutic agents when the catheters are placed
percutaneously). This reduction in the drug morbidity more

than compensates for the operative morbidity of the surgical procedure. Further, intraoperative perfusion studies enable the surgeon to position the catheter so that all of the liver parenchyma containing metastatic disease is perfused. Patient survivals of one to two years or more have been reported utilizing an implantable pump or a portable pump system (Reed, 1981).

Because similar patterns of survival follow both hepatic artery ligation and infusion chemotherapy (Table 4), a controlled trial will be needed to determine whether one or the other is superior. Hepatic artery ligation is usually followed by systemic chemotherapy. Although it is the liver metastases that are usually thought to cause the death of the patient, the median survival of patients with extra-hepatic disease is only half that of patients whose tumor is confined to the liver, whether treated by artery ligation or intra-arterial infusion. Since surgical staging of intra-abdominal disease is far more sensitive than computerized tomographic scanning, a study of infusion vs hepatic artery ligation would require laparotomy in all patients. The failure to recognize intra-abdominal disease might explain the relatively inferior survival of non-surgically staged patients who have been treated by percutaneous hepatic artery catheterization with infusion or embolization.

Resection of pulmonary metastases also prolong survival and offer a useful chance for cure when there is no disease elsewhere in the body. The best results have been seen in patients with sarcomas, particularly teenagers with osteosarcoma (Takita, 1977). Five-year survivals of 30-40 percent can be expected, survival rates being higher when single rather than multiple lesions are resected. Nevertheless, a number of patients who have had six or more lesions resected have had long-term survival.

It is our policy to perform bilateral thoracotomy through a median sternotomy when approaching the chest for metastatic disease. This permits both sides of the chest to be explored in a single procedure. Post-operative discomfort is less than that following standard thoracotomy. Since the vast majority of the metastases are subpleural, the median sternotomy approach does not limit the surgeon's ability to perform a number of wedge resections when unsuspected lesions are encountered. On occasion, recurrent

HEPATIC ARTERY LIGATION OR
INFUSION CHEMOTHERAPY FOR
HEPATIC METASTASES OF COLORECTAL CANCER

Author	Year Published	Treatment	No. of Patients	Stage	Chemo	Median Survival
Bengmark	78	HAL	15	-	HAI FU	11 mo
Evans	79	HAL	28	> 30% Ca	-	11 mo
Wallace	81	Embolized	72	-	-	11½ mo
Minton	79	HAI-pc	24	-	FU	9 mo
*Grage	79	HAI-op	30	-	FU	10 mo
Reed	81	HAI-pc	88	-	FUDR	10 mo
*Patt	81	HAI-pc	55	-	FUDR-Mit C	11 mo
Ariel	82	HAI-op	15	Asymp	FU-MTX-DDP	31 mo
*Barone	82	7 op, 8 pc	15	*	FU	8 mo

Table 4. Comparison of results of hepatic artery ligation (HAL) and hepatic artery infusion (HAI) by percutaneously (pc) or operatively (op) placed catheters. FU = 5-fluorouracil, Mit C = mitomycin C, MTX = methotrexate, FUDR = 5-fluoro-2'deoxyuridine, DDP = cis-platinum. > 30% Ca = > 30% of liver replaced by tumor. (-) = not stated. Asymp - asymptomatic patients. *Grage - control group of 31 patients received intravenous 5FU and survived a median of 13 months, *Patt noted median survival was increased to 15 months if hepatic artery occluded, *Barone noted median survival rose to 26 months if serum alkaline phosphatase was less than twice normal, and no difference between Cormed[R] (op) or Infusaid[R] (pc) pumps.

pulmonary metastases can be treated by repeat thoracotomy. We have one young osteosarcoma patient who is a long-term cure following three thoracotomies and no further adjuvant therapy.

Young men with testicular tumors, particularly following treatment with multi-drug chemotherapy, are also good candidates for resection of pulmonary metastases. In our experience, prolonged survival is also possible for patients with solitary colon, renal, and other tumors.

The pathologic fracture represents another metastatic site where the surgical oncologist has spearheaded therapy to improve the patient's quality of life. A decade ago, patients with pathologic hip fractures might have their hip fractures pinned but most were definitively treated with radiation therapy. Bone cements such as methyl-methacralate allowed more secure fixation in the face of extensive bone destruction by tumor. Thus, patients can be made pain free and functional. Of patients with lower extremity fractures, two-thirds are able to ambulate following surgical fixation, as compared to fewer than one quarter of those treated by other means (Douglass, 1976). In the upper extremity, the humerus is the most common site of fracture. Following internal fixation, two-thirds of patients with pathologic humeral fractures will have good function in their elbow and wrist and some function at the shoulder whereas not more than half of patients treated by other means will have a functional extremity. Most significant is the difference in pain relief, with nine out of ten patients treated surgically being relieved of pain at the pathologic fracture site whereas the pain is relieved in fewer than half of patients treated by other means.

Local recurrence has yielded to surgical re-resection in a number of sites. Anastomotic tumors in the pelvis following an anterior resection can occasionally be cured by posterior or total pelvic exenteration. Resection of local recurrences after esophagogastrectomy can provide, for selected patients, significant palliation. As many as half of the patients with locally recurrent sarcomas can be cured by multidisciplinary therapy (Giuliano, 1982). The development of jaundice in a patient with metastatic disease is not necessarily a terminal event. In many patients, the jaundice is found to be obstructive, responding to biliary diversion, preferably by internal hepato- or cholangiojejunostomy, but occasionally by percutaneous catheterization, providing prolonged palliation and improvement in the quality of life.

THE FUTURE OF SURGICAL ONCOLOGY

The least standardized aspect of patient care is the original surgical procedure. Since the surgical excision is often the base on which adjuvant programs are built, and since the combination of the initial surgical procedure and the adjuvant therapy will determine the overall potential for cure, it is vital that surgical oncologists undertake programs to standardize and optimize surgical procedures. An example of what can and should be done has been demonstrated by the Japanese Research Society for the Study of Gastric Cancer (Japanese Research Society for Gastric Cancer, 1981), which defined the extent of surgery and types of operation to be performed for tumors of the various parts of the stomach, documented by clinicopathologic and survival studies the appropriateness of their recommendations, and then convinced their peers to perform the procedures properly. In the United States, surgical procedures vary not only from surgeon to surgeon, but often from case to case.

The surgical oncologist must convince his colleagues of the need to document recurrent and metastatic disease (accepting biopsy rather than the laying on of hands to confirm metastases) and the need to follow patients closely for possible salvage of patients in whom there is recurrence. Because of his pivotal position in cancer care, the surgical oncologist is the best candidate to organize treatment plans involving multimodal studies, realizing that the surgical procedure may not be the first step in the therapeutic attack on the malignancy. General surgeons have proven incapable of standardizing and optimizing the treatment of cancer and the development of organized therapeutic programs based on tumor stage and tumor characteristics. Surgeons have generally abdicated their central role as treatment planners. But they are still the physicians who often see the patient first and thus offer the patient the greatest potential for cure. This gap . . . the development of treatment plans and the education of our surgical colleagues . . . is the challenge to surgical oncology today and in the future.

Adson MA, Van Heerden JA (1980). Major hepatic resections for metastatic colorectal cancer. Ann Surg 191:576.

Berjian RA, Douglass HO Jr, Nava HR (1980). The role of hepatic artery ligation and dearterialization with infusion chemotherapy in advanced malignancies in the liver. J Surg Oncol 14:379.

Broder LE, Cohen MH, Selawry OS (1977). Treatment of bronchogenic carcinoma II small cell. Cancer Treat Rep 4:219.

Douglass HO Jr (1978). Osteosarcoma: Survival gains resulting from multidisciplinary therapy. Progr Clin Cancer 7:83 New York: Grune and Stratton.

Douglass HO Jr, Shukla S, Mindell ER (1976). Treatment of pathologic fractures of long bones excluding those due to breast cancer. J Bone Joint Surg 58A:1055.

Evans JT (1979). Hepatic artery ligation in hepatic metastases from colon and rectal malignancies. Dis Colon Rectum 22:370.

Foster JH (1978). Resection of metastatic cancer from the liver. Contemporary Surg 12:26.

Gastrointestinal Tumor Study Group (Douglass HO Jr, Stablein DM) (1982). Controlled trial of adjuvant chemotherapy following curative resection for gastric cancer. Cancer 49:1116.

Giuliano AE, Eilber FR, Morton DL (1982). The management of locally recurrent soft tissue sarcoma. Ann Surg 196:87.

Japanese Research Society for Gastric Cancer (1981 In English). The general rules for the gastric cancer study in surgery and pathology. Part I clinical classification. Jpn J Surg 11:127.

Reed ML, Vaitkevicius VK, Al-Sarraf M, Vaughn CB, Singhaktowinta A, Sexon-Porte M, Izbicki R, Baker LE, Straatsma GW (1981). The practicality of chronic hepatic artery infusion therapy of primary and metastatic malignancies. Ten-year results of 124 patients in a prospective protocol. Cancer 47:402.

Takita H, Merrin C, Didolkar MS, Douglass HO Jr, Edgerton F (1977). The surgical management of multiple lung metastases. Ann Thoracic Surg 24:359.

13th International Cancer Congress, Part A
Current Perspectives in Cancer, pages 47-69
© **1983 Alan R. Liss, Inc., 150 Fifth Avenue, New York, NY 10011**

ADVANCES IN CANCER THERAPEUTICS: CHEMOTHERAPY

Vincent T. DeVita, Jr., M.D.

National Cancer Institute

Bethesda, Maryland 20205

Abstract

Tumor mass negatively influences the outcome of surgery and radiotherapy by its influence on invasiveness and the propensity to metastasize before local treatment is applied. Tumor mass negatively affects the outcome of cancer chemotherapy in a manner quite different from the way in which it does surgery or radiotherapy. Cancer chemotherapy fails because cells develop resistance to anti-cancer drugs. Conceptually, there are two types of resistance both of which are mass related: temporary resistance (due to pharmacologic sanctuaries or altered cell kinetics) or permanent resistance (mutant lines developing specific and permanent resistance to one or more cancer drugs). Based on somatic mutation theory, it now appears that resistant mutants arise spontaneously early in the natural history of cancers, and the likelihood of a resistant line developing appears closely related to cell number, such that one or more resistant lines are likely present before most human malignancies become clinically evident. The development of permanent resistance more precisely accounts for the invariable inverse relationship between cell number and curability by drugs and the greater effectiveness of combination chemotherapy over single agents. New information on common pathways of drug resistance appears exploitable using tools available today or on the horizon. While this revolution in our understanding of resistance to chemotherapy is occurring, the information on the role of oncogenes in the origin of human cancer offers a new paradigm for cancer diagnosis, prevention and treatment in the 1980s. In 1980 we estimate that approximately 50,000 patients in the U.S. per year are curable due to chemotherapy used alone or in combination with surgery and/or radiotherapy.

Milestones in Cancer Treatment

Although good data for the period from 1900 to 1950 are scarce, the survival rates of cancer patients in the U.S. appeared to increase from near 0 in 1900 to approximately 30 percent in the 1950s with the use of surgery alone. Although radiotherapy was available during this period, the equipment was difficult to use and radiotherapy did not have a large impact on national survival until later. Since then, the trend in cancer surgery has been from the more radical to the more conservative surgical procedures as other effective ways of complementing surgery have become available for treatment of the primary tumor. But the most radical recent departure in cancer surgery has been the introduction of the surgical treatment of metastases in patients with advanced cancer. According to 1980 data (DeVita VT, Henney JE, Hubbard SM, 1981) in the U.S.A., approximately 220,000 patients are curable by surgery alone.

With the introduction of cobalt radiotherapy in 1952 and the linear accelerator in 1957, it became possible to give wide-field radiotherapy with less toxicity. Concomitant with the training of some 1,500 radiotherapists, radiotherapy has become a major tool, not only for cure but palliation of patients with cancer. The literature of the 1920s and 30s was replete with expressions of alarm about toxicity from radiotherapy to the extent of suggesting it was too toxic for use in cancer treatment and should be discarded as a treatment modality. This hasty judgment would indeed have deprived many cancer patients of what is today a very effective form of treatment. The introduction of mega and super-voltage radiotherapy had a measurable impact on five-year survival rates for a numerous cancers between 1955 and 1970. Today, approximately 90,000 patients a year in the U.S. are curable using radiotherapy alone or in combination with other modalities.

The effective use of chemotherapy to treat human cancers awaited the demonstration that rodents with cancer could be cured by drugs. Then it remained to be shown that drugs could cure spontaneous cancers in humans and this was satisfactorily done by 1970. Some cancer cells hid in sanctuaries and, at first, this was thought to be the main reason for failure of drugs to cure greater numbers of patients. Effective sanctuary therapy proved to be an important advance in the treatment of acute lymphocytic leukemia of childhood where the cure rate is substantially reduced if treatment of the central nervous system is not carried out. However, the most important recent milestone in cancer chemotherapy is the use of chemotherapy in conjunction with surgery and radiotherapy -- so-called combined modality treatment which is often the first approach to managing patients with cancer today. Combined modality treatment has led to a greater number of live, intact persons who have had cancer and, for the first time in this century, has resulted in reduction of age- and disease-specific national mortality in those diseases where successful treatments have been developed (DeVita VT, Henney JE, Weiss RB, 1980; DeVita VT, Henney JE, Hubbard SM, 1981; Weiss RB, DeVita VT, 1979; Weiss RB, Henney JE, DeVita VT, 1981). Today the NCI's Surveillance, Epidemiology, End-Results (SEER) program indicates that the relative survival rates (RSR) or all cancers treated between 1973 and 1978 is 45 percent. This represents an increase of 12 percent over the RSR derived from a different data base covering the period from 1969 to 1973. Approximately 50,000 of the patients successfully treated owe their lives to chemotherapy alone or in concert with combined modality programs developed since chemotherapy was effectively introduced as a treatment option in the late 1950s. Table 1 illustrates the evolution of cancer chemotherapy since the early part of this century. The major opportunity in the chemotherapy arena in the 1980s appears to be the possibility of a solution of the problem of drug resistance. This has been the major roadblock to the successful use of chemotherapy in patients with widespread metastatic disease. The development of drug resistance now appears related to tumor mass in ways not previously appreciated.

The relationship of tumor mass to prognosis is not a new subject, especially for surgeons. Tables 2 and 3 illustrate these points by simply using data on breast cancer from the National Surgical Adjuvant Breast Project and Milan studies as examples (Fisher B, Slack NM, Bross IDJ, 1969; Santoro A, Bonnadonna G, Veronesi U, 1978). Tumor size influences the likelihood of nodal involvement, which in turn influences curability by surgery (Table 2). Table 3 extends this point further by showing the relationship of the degree of nodal involvement from these two studies to the relapse rate. No matter what the approach to treating the cancer, or the type

of cancer, the greater the tumor mass, the lower the likelihood of cure. In the example cited above, however, mass
influences prognosis primarily through its influence on the
invasiveness of the tumor and its tendency to metastasize.

Table 1. PHASES IN THE DEVELOPMENT OF CANCER CHEMOTHERAPY

---

1. The antibacterial and antimalarial models (1935-1945)
2. The period of total empiricism (1945-1960)
    ° Single-agent treatment
    ° Abortive attempts at combination chemotherapy
3. The principles of cancer chemotherapy (1960-1975)
    ° The fatal single cell
    ° Fractional kill
    ° Cell kinetics and temporary resistance
    ° The invariable inverse relationship between cell
      number and curability
    ° Successful use of combination chemotherapy
4. Widespread application of chemotherapy and effects on
    national mortality (1970 to present)
5. Widespread application of chemotherapy as adjuvant to
    surgery and radiotherapy (1974 to present)
6. The "barrier" (1975 to 1979)
7. Drug resistance and tumor mass; a new understanding
    (1980--)
8. The antibacterial and antimalarial model revisited
    (1935 to present)

Table 2. RELATIONSHIP OF TUMOR SIZE AND NODAL STATUS TO
          DISEASE-FREE SURVIVAL AT FIVE YEARS*

	Tumor Size, cm						
	<1	1-2	2-3	3-4	4-5	5-6	>6
Number of patients	19	138	234	217	146	132	162
Percent with positive nodes	26	43	43	57	51	67	64
Percent of patients with positive nodes free of disease	80	47	49	36	36	28	16

*Fisher et al. 1,049 patients

Table 3.   EFFECT OF LYMPH NODE INVOLVEMENT ON RECURRENCE OF
BREAST CANCER AFTER MASTECTOMY (PREMENOPAUSAL AND
POSTMENOPAUSAL WOMEN)

Axillary node status			Relapse Rate	
	18 mo*	3 yr†	5 yr	10 yr
Negative	5	15	18*;21†	24*;28†
1-3 positive	16	40	50*;54†	65*;67†
>4 positive	44	65	79*;74†	86*;84†
All patients	18	35	40*;44†	50*;53†

*NSABP -- USA. Fisher et al.
†Instituto Nazionale Tumori, Milan. Valagussa et al.

Around 1960 Skipper and his colleagues elucidated principles of cancer chemotherapy that also related successful
treatment to cell number in rodent malignancies disseminated
at the time of treatment. These were: (a) the reaffirmation
of the observation of Furth and Kahn, first made in 1937,
that a single malignant cell could grow to a lethal number
of cells and overwhelm the host (Furth J, Kahn MC, 1937),
(b) that tumor growth followed Gompertzian growth kinetics;
exponential growth was followed by exponential retardation
of growth as the body burden of tumor increased, (c) the
killing effect of drugs was a logarithmic function, that
is, a given dose killed a constant fraction of cells, regard-
less of the number present at the start and (d), that there
was an invariable inverse relationship between cell number
and curability by chemotherapy. Presumably then, anti-cancer
drugs could cure if the dose of drug were increased to increase the fractional kill or if the treatment were started
while the number of malignant cells present was small enough
so that all malignant cells could be destroyed (Skipper HE,
1978; Skipper HE, Schabel FM, Wilcox WS, 1964). By treating
mice bearing leukemia L1210 armed only with a knowledge of
tumor volume doubling times, Skipper and his colleagues
back-extrapolated from prolongation of survival to estimate
the number of cells killed per treatment. Using these kinds
of experiments, doses and schedules that reduced the L1210
leukemic population maximally were developed, eradicating
the final potentially lethal cell. This observation had an
important impact on the design of clinical protocols in the
early 1960s. Mice bearing L1210 leukemia die with a body
burden of about 10^9 cells. Therapies effective at a body

burden of 10^5 often failed at 10^9 cells. In part this was perceived to be a limitation of the steep dose response curve of cytotoxic drugs and combination chemotherapy was employed to maximize cell kill and reduce the body burden of cells, in doses and schedules that were not fatal to the mouse. These experiments were mimicked in the clinics with some stunning successes (DeVita VT, 1978). As can be seen in Table 1, by the mid-1970s, a plateau in the effectiveness of chemotherapy that represented resistance to treatment was reached.

For convenience, resistance to cancer chemotherapy can be examined as two separate categories: temporary and permanent. Temporary resistance can be divided further into two separate problems (Table 4): First, resistance due to physiologic barriers (DeVita VT, 1982), the inability of an effective drug, or its metabolite, to reach the viable cancer cell because a physiological barrier prevents diffusion of the active moiety of the drug to the site occupied by the cell, or because of differences in drug metabolism between rodents and humans. The second problem is the inability of a drug to kill cancer cells because changes in the growth characteristics of the tumor decrease its vulnerability to the effects of drugs.

Table 4.   CAUSES OF TEMPORARY RESISTANCE TO CANCER
            CHEMOTHERAPY

1. Pharmacologic sanctuaries
   ° Inaccessible compartments
   ° Blood supply and diffusion
   ° Cell cycle phase specificity of "active" drugs

2. Alteration in cell kinetics
   ° Growth fraction decreases with increasing tumor mass
   ° Cells enter resting phase but remain viable
   ° Cell-shedding increases with increase in size of tumor
   ° Growth fraction influenced by proximity to blood supply

Pharmacologic sanctuaries proved to be real enough and very early in the 1960s studies of such sanctuaries in patients with leukemia and the development of subsequent special approaches to their treatment, led to the improvement in the durability of remissions in this disease. It was soon clear, however, that even in acute lymphatic leukemia, the majority

of relapses occurred not because cells were in physiologic
compartments inaccessible to drugs or to differences in activa-
tion and deactivation of drugs. As pharmacologic sanctuaries
ceased to be viewed as the major reason for treatment failure,
attention shifted to the other major form of temporary resistance, i.e., differences in growth characteristics of tumor,
the study of cell kinetics (DeVita VT, 1971).

Part of the failure to cure mice with large volumes of
tumor was perceived to be related to the slowing of the tumor
doubling times at large tumor volumes. Since human tumors
were often diagnosed when patients had a large body burden of
cancer (greater than 10^{10} cells), the failure to achieve
effects in humans comparable to that in rodents was attributed to the potential kinetic differences between mouse and
human cancers and/or similarities between the growth kinetics
of normal human tissues and its respective cancer, and other
normal target tissue such as bone marrow and the gastrointestinal crypt cells (DeVita VT, 1971; DeVita VT, Schein
PS, 1973). The study of tumor cell kinetics entered its
descriptive phase in 1959, facilitated by the availability of
tritiated thymidine which made it possible to label cells syn-
thesizing DNA and follow them through their life cycles, to
determine cell cycle times (Young RC, DeVita VT, 1970), duration of phases of the cell cycle and the proportion of a
population cycling (the growth fraction) (Mendelsohn ML,
1962). What followed was a series of studies to determine
the precise cell kinetic parameters of L1210 at various tumor
volumes (DeVita VT 1971; Yankee RA, DeVita VT, Perry S,
1968; Young RC, DeVita VT, Perry S, 1969), normal mouse
marrow (DeVita VT, 1971), the kinetics of other rodent tumors
(Simpson-Herren L, Sanford AH, Holmquist JP, 1976; Simpson-
Herren L, Springer TA, Sanford AH, Holmquist JP, 1977; Steel
GG, Stephens TC, 1979) and the eventual translation of the
tedious techniques required to do these studies in human
tumors and comparable human target tissues (Young RC, DeVita
VT, 1970).

The data can be summarized as follows: In both humans
and rodents, only small differences between the cell cycle
time of a normal and cancerous cell of the same organ could
be identified. In other words, cancer cells did not divide
more rapidly than did normal cells. Cancers grew by progres-
sive steady expansion due to differences in growth fraction
between cancerous and normal tissue (Steel GG, 1979; Steel
GG, Stephens TC, 1979). In mice and men, as tumor volume

increased, growth fraction (and labelling index) decreased. Normal target tissue growth characteristics (bone marrow) varied in different species (mice and men) but could be measured and its behavior was characteristically consistent (DeVita VT, 1971). Then chemotherapy cycles could be designed around the vulnerable phases of regrowth of normal target tissue.

As tumors grew larger, they outstripped their blood supply, and distance from blood vessels was a cause of reduction in the growth fraction (Tannock, I, 1978). Doubling time, as used in Skipper's early classic studies (Skipper HE, Schabel, FM, Wilcox WS, 1964), proved to be an inaccurate reflection of the actual rate of tumor expansion of most solid rodent and human tumors because cell loss during growth varied considerably from tumor to tumor. As tumor mass increased, cell loss increased. A tumor with a slow doubling time could have a high growth fraction and double slowly due to extensive cell loss. The clinical counterpart to cell loss is, of course, the potential for metastasis if shed cells are viable. Micrometastases were shown to have higher labelling indices than did larger tumor masses (Simpson-Herren L, Springer TA, Sanford AH, Holmquist JP, 1977) and, in some tumors, removal of the primary tumor led to an increase in the labelling index of the metastatic deposits (Gunduz N, Fisher B, Saffer EA, 1979). These observations have been directly responsible for the enthusiasm in applying chemotherapy as an adjuvant to surgery or radiotherapy, since it was assumed that small amounts of residual tumors should be kinetically more vulnerable to drugs and gentler therapy could achieve easy cures. The use of drugs to treat micrometastases in rodents after excision of the primary tumor yielded positive results, if not as positive as anticipated at first. (Schabel, FM, 1975). The data in Figure 1 illustrate the problem facing clinical oncologists. Even at the time of diagnosis, most cancers have completed 32 doublings and are near the end of their life cycle. These kinds of data led to attempts to overcome kinetic forms of temporary resistance by using combination chemotherapy which met with some considerable success. Dose, dose-rate, and scheduling proved to be important variables in clinical protocols. The use of cell-cycle-specific drugs (active during the DNA synthetic period) together or alternating with cycle-phase nonspecific drugs, and intermittent cycles of chemotherapy was viewed as integral to the success of combination chemotherapy. Such approaches clearly limited

.ethal injury to normal target tissue due to large toxic
loses of individual drugs and also avoided retreatment during
;he recovery phase of bone marrow cells. Most clinical com-
)inations of drugs are given on 28-day schedules, an interval
vhich has been shown to allow for bone marrow recovery before
i second cycle of treatment was begun (DeVita VT, 1982;
)eVita, Schein PS, 1973; DeVita VT, Simon RM, Hubbard SM,
foung, RRC, Berard CW, Moxley JH, Frei E, Carbone PP,
Janellos GP, 1980).

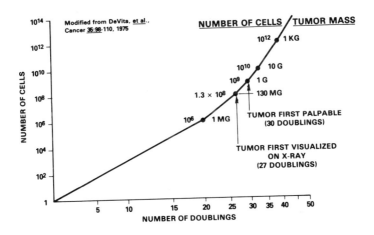

Fig. 1. The life cycle of human cancers relating clinical
events to the number of cells and population doublings.

     Some puzzling observations were made in clinical studies
in the mid 1970s. First, only combinations of drugs known to
be individually effective worked (DeVita VT, Schein PS, 1973;
DeVita VT, Henney JE, Weiss RB, 1980). Second, while complete
remissions were achieved in dozens of tumor types, usually a
significant fraction of patients who had achieved complete
remission relapsed and would fail to respond satisfactorily
to any further treatment. It was usually not possible to
predict which patients would relapse, based on any known
clinical characteristics. Tumor volume itself was not as

good a predictor of curability in the clinic as one would
have expected on the basis of available cell kinetic data.
Some patients with massive amounts of certain kinds of
cancer achieved permanent remission with drug combinations
(such as those with Stage IV diffuse histiocytic lymphoma,
Hodgkin's disease, acute leukemia, testicular carcinomas,
etc.) or even single agents (Burkitt's lymphoma and choriocarcinoma). In some cases, drug combinations as adjuvants to
surgery or radiotherapy were no more effective than the same
treatment in patients with advanced disease (Weiss RB,
DeVita VT, 1979). An extraordinary observation had also
been largely overlooked and unexplained: Normal target tissue
never developed resistance to chemotherapy.

Drug Resistance and Tumor Mass; A New Understanding

In 1979 Goldie and Coldman (Goldie JH, Coldman AJ,
Gudauskas GA, 1982) reexamined the work of Luria and Delbruck
for its relevance to cancer chemotherapy. Ample evidence
existed in mammalian cell systems that spontaneous and permanent mutation to phenotypic drug resistance could occur
as an intrinsic property of genetically unstable rapidly
growing malignant cell lines relative to normal regenerating
tissue (Baker RM, Ling VM; Heppner GH, Dexter DL, DeNucci T,
Miller FR, Calabresi P, 1978; Law LW, 1952; Ling VM, 1975;
Ling VM, 1982; Simonovich L, 1976). The failure of bone
marrow tissue to develop resistance to anti-cancer drugs
suggests that most mammalian cells perhaps including all
cancer cells, start out sensitive to the toxic effects of
these drugs. In patients whose tumor, first sensitive to
chemotherapy, became progressively more resistant to treatment and ultimately overwhelmed the host, marrow toxicity
is always a concomitant of re-exposure to the increasingly
ineffective drugs. Goldie and Coldman developed a mathematical model which related curability to the time of appearance of a singly or doubly resistant cell line. Assuming
a mutation rate approximating the natural mutation frequency,
their model predicted that there is a variation in size of
the resistant fraction in tumors of the same size and type,
depending on the value of the mutation rate and the point at
which a mutation develops. Given such assumptions, the
proportion of resistant cells in any given mass is likely to
be small and the initial response to a treatment should not
be influenced by the number of resistant cells. (In a clinic
this means that a complete remission could be attained even
if a resistant cell line were present.) Failure to achieve a

significant clinical response would occur only if the proportion of resistant cells exceeded 50 percent of the tumor mass. Failure to cure, (relapse from a complete remission) would, however, be directly dependent on the presence or absence of doubly resistant cell lines. Some experimental data using the Goldie-Coldman assumptions have been plotted by Skipper and are shown in Figures 2 and 3 for cyclophosphamide and arabinosyl cytosine. Using the same dose and schedule for each drug, the curability of the rodent tumor diminishes as tumor cell number increases between 10^5 and 10^8 cells, fitting the curve E for a mutation rate of approximately 10^{-7}.

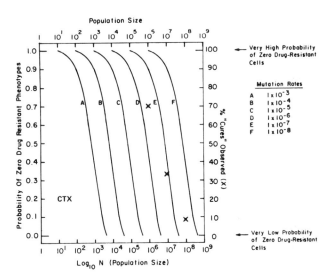

Fig. 2. Plots based on Goldie-Coldman model. Effects of increasing population size on the ability of cyclophosphamide to cure. Cure rate (x) drops from 70 to less than 10 percent as population increases from 10^6 to 10^8 cells fitting the curve depicting a mutation rate of 10^{-7} (curve E).

Recently, Goldie and Coldman have published on a computer-assisted program to develop strategies for managing treatable cancers with existing chemotherapy (Goldie JH, Coldman AJ, Gudauskas GA, 1982). Their basic assumption is that tumors are curable by chemotherapy if no permanently resistant cell lines

are present. But curability diminishes rapidly with the appearance of a single resistant line, if only one effective
therapy (T_1) is available, or with the appearance of a doubly
resistant line, if two equally effective therapies are available. Two equally effective therapies (T_1 and T_2) can be
either two single agents or two equally effective combinations
of noncross-resistant drugs. For the purposes of their model,
they make certain clinically and experimentally realistic
assumptions: (a) That cell-kill is a logarithmic function.
(b) That the rate of spontaneous mutation toward resistance
occurs at about the natural frequency of 10^{-5} or 10^{-6}.
(c) That mutation to resistance is a stepwise function from
sensitivity to resistance to the first treatment (R_1) to
resistance to the second treatment with the appearance of a
doubly resistant line (R_{1-2}). The model approximates
characteristics of some human cancers that are already known

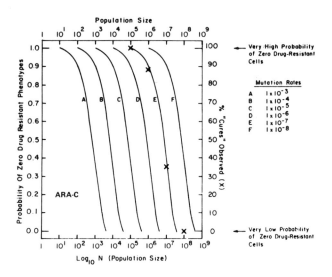

Fig. 3. Plot based on Goldie-Coldman model. Effects of
increasing population size on the ability of arabinosyl cytosine to cure. Cure rate (x) decreases from near 100 percent at
about 10^5 cells to zero as population size increases from 10^5
to 10^8 along line E, depicting a mutation rate of 10^{-7}.

to be curable to some extent by chemotherapy, (durable complete remissions attained in some fraction of patients when the tumor is clinically evident (mass $\pm\ 10^{10}$ cells); a doubling times of 36 days and a log kill per treatment of 2, with treatment intervals of 21 days). It further assumes two treatments of equal efficacy which cannot be given simultaneously. Under such circumstances, the proportion of cells resistant to T_1 or T_2 in a mass of 10^{10} cells is small and will not affect initial response rate. The maximal cure rate predicted in the model tumor described is about 64 percent. Selection of the wrong strategy will reduce the cure rate from this maximal level to some lower level. Their model predicts that alternating cycles of treatment (T_1, T_2, T_1, T_2, T_1, T_2) would be superior to sequential use of T_1 and T_2 (T_1, T_1, T_1, T_1, T_2, T_2, T_2, etc.) because of the propensity for the latter approach to allow development and regrowth of a doubly resistant line. Continued used of T_1, although it will result in a clinical remission, will allow a cell line resistant to T_1 to mutate to R_{1-2} and, is ultimately doomed to failure by the eventual overgrowth of line R_{1-2} resistant to both T_1 and T_2. Readers are referred to their two recent excellent publications on this subject for detailed illustrations of these treatment strategies (Goldie JH, Coldman AJ, Gudauskas GA, 1982; Goldie, JH, Coldman AJ, 1979). To improve results of drug treatment at the clinical level using their model, it should be reemphasized that two equally effective combinations of drugs are required. These conditions are met clinically in only a few human tumors today such as acute lymphocytic leukemia, Hodgkin's disease and diffuse histiocytic lymphoma (DeVita VT, Henney JE, Hubbard SM, 1981). In Hodgkin's disease, alternating cycles of MOPP and the non-cross-resistant combination ABVD appear superior to MOPP alone in some categories of disease (Santoro A, Bonnadonna G, Bonfante V, Valagussa P, 1982) and in diffuse histiocytic lymphoma, alternating MOPP with the ProMACE combination may be superior to MOPP alone (Fisher RI, DeVita VT, Hubbard SM, Jaffe Es, Cossman J, Wesley R, Chabner BA, Young RC, 1982). All of these experiments were designed intuitively by clinicians. The Goldie-Coldman model, however, may provide a prospective way of designing their use in treatment protocols when other variables are added to the data set. Additional assumptoms of their model critical to the successful application of this strategy may not be consistent with what actually happens under clinical circumstances, such as the requirement for similar growth characteristics in multiple metastatic sites of the same tumor in the same or in different patients, and equivalent log kill for each treatment program. These and other variables will make the actual development of such strategies more complicated.

There are three major clinical implications of the Goldie-Coldman hypothesis: (a) First and foremost, these data suggest a reason why chemotherapy may not be much more effective in the adjuvant setting than in patients with clinically evident tumors, even though the growth characteristics of micrometa-vulnerable to drug treatment (DeVita VT, Schein PS, 1973; Frei E, Jaffe AN, Gero N, 1978; Salmon SE, 1977; Schabel FM, 1975; Weiss RB, DeVita VT, 1979). (b) Time-to-first-drug-treatment may be more important than had been appreciated previously. Thus, if a resistant line can develop spontane-ously in weeks at a subclinical tumor cell number, adjuvant therapy should be started as soon as possible. Adjuvant studies with breast cancer suggest that even a short delay in starting chemotherapy may have an important negative influence on outcome (Weiss RB, Henney JE, DeVita VT, 1981). (c) Attempts to improve responses to chemotherapy by "debulking" operations to reduce tumor mass and favorably alter cell kinetic characteristics have not been successful in increasing cure rate and, according to the Goldie-Coldman hypothesis, could not be expected to be successful. Since mutation toward resistance is mass related, patients with large masses of cancer prior to "debulking" already have a a high likelihood of having developed at least one and probably more than one resistant cell line. If these lines have metastasized widely prior to reductive surgery, reducing the mass, while it may improve response to chemotherapy, is not likely to improve curability unless the resistant lines in large tumor masses have little propensity to metastasize.

Goldie and Coldman's theory suggests a variation in muta-tion rate even in tumors of the same type but, more importantly, it may also explain the wide variance in response to drugs of tumors originating from different organs. For example, if spontaneous development of phenotypic resistance is a common phenomenon in the clinic, current clinical data suggest that tumors of B-cell origin probably have a lower inherent tendency than more common visceral cancers to develop resistant lines, even when massive amounts of tumor are present. For example, Burkitt's lymphoma, a tumor of follicular center B-cells, is curable by the single drug cyclophosphamide, even in advanced stages (DeVita VT, Henney JE, Hubbard SM, 1981). In other indolent lymphomas of B-cell origin, such as the nodular, poorly differentiated lymphocytic lymphomas (NPDL), patients respond well to single agent chemotherapy and can often be retreated with the same drug even after relapsing several times. Treatment results are no better with combination chemotherapy, and no known drug combination at tolerable dose levels will cure patients with NPDL (Longo DL, Young RC, DeVita VT, 1982). This tumor has been shown to have growth characteristics similar to normal B-lymphocytes (Hanson H, Koziner B, Clarkson B, 1981). Such data suggest relative genetic stability in NPDL lines with little tendency to mutation toward phenotypic resistance to available drugs while in the "near normal" nodular phase. When NPDL evolves to the diffuse large-celled lymphomas (diffuse histiocytic lymphomas [DHL]), as they have been shown to do with some frequency (Hubbard SM, Chabner BA, DeVita VT, Simon R, Berard CW, Jones RB, Garvin AJ, Canellos GP, Osborne GK, Young, RC, 1982), it is curable by drugs, but combination chemotherapy is an absolute requirement for cure (DeVita VT, 1981). The DHL that evolves from NPDL is now known to derive from the same monoclonal B-cell line. This suggests that increasing genetic instability that is associated with development of phenotypic resistance occurs as the tumor evolves to a less differentiated, more rapidly growing cell line. Combination chemotherapy, when it works in DHL, will also cure patients with massive amounts of tumor, suggesting that the mutation rate is still relatively low, so that a single treatment program with four drugs covers the resistant lines. Hodgkin's disease, a tumor of probable macrophage origin, is curable by combination chemotherapy, but not by single drugs (DeVita VT, Lewis BJ, Rozencweig M, Muggia FM, 1978). Reed-Sternberg cells and their mononuclear variants make up only a small proportion of the palpable tumor masses in Hodgkin's disease, and thus the malignant cell population in tumor masses of any given strain are in the minority.

The mutation rate in the malignant cell line may also be relatively low; spontaneous mutation rates in some tumors may also vary, depending on the etiologic factor responsible for the tumor. The circumstances surrounding the origin of tumors like carcinoma of the lung may be the reverse of B-cell tumors and Hodgkin's disease. If lung cancer is due to exposure to the multiple carcinogenic chemicals in cigarette smoke, then the spontaneous mutation rate may higher under the pressure of these mutagenic materials than the natural frequency. Numerous drug resistant lines may be present before tumors are even clinically evident and account for the failure of chemotherapy to work against this disease.

There are implications for the design of future chemotherapy adjuvant trials in these data: First, combination chemotherapy rather than single agent therapy is a likely requirement for adjuvant chemotherapy programs as it is for most of the successful treatment programs for patients with clinically evident disease. Second, adjuvant chemotherapy is not likely to be effective unless the intensity of treatment of micrometastases is at least commensurate with that used for clinically evident disease of the same tumor type. Third, drugs that produce partial responses in patients with clinically evident disease should not necessarily be expected to produce better results (cures) in the adjuvant setting, as has been shown by most studies of patients with colon cancer. Fourth, the duration of treatment may not need to be as lengthy as was thought in the past if the multiplicity of drugs and the intensity of their administration is sufficient to eradicate relatively small numbers of resistant tumor cells. In fact, a lengthy period of adjuvant therapy could accelerate the growth of a resistant population by enhancing its mutation rate. And finally, preoperative chemotherapy, as has been used in some studies in patients with head and neck cancer, may provide important clues to the usefulness of a drug program that is proposed for use in the post-surgical or post-radiotherapeutic phase of treatment.

The Spontaneous Development of Phenotypic Resistance in Mammalian Cells

Inherent in the Goldie-Coldman model is the assumption that phenotypic resistance to chemotherapy is a spontaneous phenomenon which occurs prior to exposure to chemotherapy. If so, successful chemotherapy (complete remission) followed by relapse and resistance to further treatment is the result of the expression of the growth and overpopulation of a resistant line present at the time treatment was started. That this was the mechanism of bacterial resistance to phage was quite clearly established by Luria and Delbruck in 1943 (Luria SE, Delbruck M, 1943). There is now considerable evidence that such is the case for malignant mammalian cells as well. This subject has been reviewed recently in detail by Ling (Baker RM, Ling V, 1978). While epigenetic phenomena may occur after exposure to anticancer drugs that partially or permanently alter the ability of the cells to respond to drugs, such changes may and could have, by now, been overcome by pharmacologic or biochemical modulation, some of which was considered even in the earliest of drug combination studies (DeVita VT, 1978).

The criteria for the genetic origin of drug resistant phenotypes are shown are Table 5. Examples that meet all or most of these criteria exist and result in three major mechanisms of drug resistance: overproduction of the drug target (gene amplification) (Schimke RT, Kaufman RJ, Alt FW, Kellems RF, 1978); altered interaction of the drug with its target; and reduced membrane permeability to drugs. The first two mechanisms often result in specific resistance to a single agent, most often an antimetabolite. Recently, an important observation relating to the latter mechanism has been reported by Ling (Ling V, 1975; Ling V, 1978; Ling V, 1982). He and his colleagues have identified a resistant line which expresses resistance to multiple classes of unrelated anti-tumor

Table 5. EVIDENCE FOR GENETIC ORIGIN OF DRUG-RESISTANT PHENOTYPE

1. Stably inherited in the absence of selection.
2. Spontaneously generated; mutation rate consistent with natural populations.
3. Frequency increased by mutagens.
4. An altered gene product can be demonstrated
5. An altered gene can be demonstrated at the DNA level.

agents. Apparently, this line was spontaneously generated and grows selectively in the presence of colchicine. There are several important points to be emphasized here: first, multi-drug resistance in a single line has been observed before, but not characterized as a result of a single genetic change (Heppner GH, Dexter DL, DeNucci T, Miller FR, Calabresi P, 1978; Salles B, Charcosset Y-V, Jacquemin-Sablon A, 1982). Second, while the observation has been made in Chinese hamster ovary cells, it has been extended to include rodent tumors and even human tumors (Ling V, 1982). Third, a single surface protein is associated with the genetic change (the P-glyco-protein) and is apparently associated with altered capacity of the cells to transport a variety of unrelated chemical structures across the membrane. The higher the concentration of surface protein, the greater the degree of resistance. These lines are most resistant to complex chemicals derived from either plants or microbia. The resistance develops as a two-step process. Of singular importance, is that the presence of the P-glycoprotein can be detected and monitored by specific antibody.

When pleiotropic resistance develops, collateral sensitivity to other classes of anti-cancer drugs and hormones appears (Ling V, 1982). Collateral sensitivity has been observed for a number of years but, has heretofore not been exploitable clinically (Brockman RW, 1974; Hutchison DJ, Schmid FA, 1973). While the range and degree of resistance in the pleiotropic resistant phenotype varies, the drugs affected are usually in classes most useful in cancer treatment today, such as the anthracyclines (adriamycin and daunorubicin) and the vinca alkaloids (vinblastine and vincristine), as well as some alkylating agents. Coupled with the Goldie-Coldman hypothesis, the observation of Ling et al. may prove to be of seminal importance to overcoming the problem of resistance to cancer chemotherapy. It now appears likely that the major reason for failure of cancer chemotherapy can be attributed to cancer cells backing away from the effects of current treatment programs in a series of predictable and therefore potentially exploitable steps.

A Paralogical Leap to a Different Paradigm

While this exciting revolution in our thinking about the development of drug resistance is taking place, a revolution of a different sort is in progress. Oncogenes identified in RNA tumor viruses over the past decade-and-a-half, have now been found to have normal cellular homologs in vertebrates (Coffin JM, Varumus HE, Bishop JM, Essex M, Harcy WD, Martin GS, Rosenberg NE, Scolnick EM, Weinberg RA, Boft PK, 1981; Der CJ, Krontieris TG, Cooper JM, 1982). This is an extraordinary observation. Recent data from DNA transfection experiments (the transfer of DNA from one cell to another) has shown that fragments of DNA from human colon, bladder, and other types of cancer can transform NIH 3T3 fibroblast cell lines, and these DNA fragments are, in some cases, homologous to the viral oncogenes. Some 17 such oncogenes have now been identified. It is at least a reasonable hypothesis that cancer is caused by an overdose of these genes, probably working through an overdose of the gene product itself. Since these genes appear to exist in normal tissue, the gene product itself may have a normal function in the development of vertebrates. Great excitement surrounds research on the identification of the function of these gene products. A somewhat paralogical leap in thinking in the 1980s could be the convergence of diagnosis, prevention, and treatment focused exclusively on the action of these gene products. If, in fact, cancer is caused by an excess production of one or more

of these gene products, it might be possible to identify before-
hand individuals who are destined to develop cancer. Having
done this, it remains to prevent the development of these
cancer. Promoters and anti-promoters may be working through
the mechanism which is related somehow to the function of
oncogenes. Knowing the function of a gene product that causes
a cell to become malignant could also allow us to identify a
way of interfering with the growth of the malignancy after it
has developed. In other words, it may be possible to tailor
more specific forms of treatment for patients who present with
metastatic disease.

Conclusions

In conclusion, data generated by the expanded research
effort in the Cancer Program indicate we have much to be opti-
mistic about in our struggle against this dread disease during
the coming decade. Cancers are, after all chronic illnesses.
Cancers, although frequently fatal, appear to be the most
curable group of chronic diseases in the U.S.A. today. This
paper emphasizes changes in treatment, primarily chemotherapy.
Much evidence not reviewed here indicates that cancer may
also be the most preventable group of chronic diseases. The
National Cancer Program is now in a position to set and monitor
national goals, both in prevention and treatment of specific
cancers.

References

Baker RM, Ling V (1978). Numbering mutants of mammalian cells
in culture In: Korn, ED, (ed) " Methods in Membrane Biology,"
New York: Plenum Press, p. 337.

Brockman RW (1974). Mechanisms of resistance. In: Sartorelli
AC, Johns DG, (eds.) "Antineoplastic and Immunosuppressive
Agents," Berlin, Germany, Springer-Verlag, p. 354.

Coffin JM, Varumus HE, Bishop JM, Essex M, Harcy, WD Jr, Martin
GS, Rosenberg, NE, Scolnick EM, Weinberg RA, Boft PK (1981).
Proposal for naming the host cell-derived inserts in retro-
virus genomes. J Virol 40:953.

Der CJ, Krontieris TG, Cooper JM (1982). Transforming genes of
human bladder and lung carcinoma cell lines are homologous
to the ras genes of Harvey and Kirsten sarc viruses. Proc
Natl Acad Sci USA 79:3637.

DeVita VT Jr (1982). The relationship between tumor mass and
resistance to chemotherapy: implications for surgical adjuvant treatment of cancer. Cancer (in press).

DeVita VT (1971). Cell kinetics and the chemotherapy of cancer. Cancer Chemother Rep 3(2)(1):23.

DeVita VT, Schein PS (1973). The use of drugs in combination for the treatment of cancer: Rationale and results. N Engl J Med 288(19):998.

DeVita VT (1978). The evolution of therapeutic research in cancer. N Engl J Med 298(16):907.

DeVita VT, Lewis BJ, Rozencweig M, Muggia FM (1978). The chemotherapy of Hodgkin's disease: Past experiences and future directions. Cancer 42(2):979.

DeVita VT, Simon RM, Hubbard SM, Young RC, Berard CW, Moxley JH III, Frei E III, Carbone PP, Canellos GP (1980). Curability of advanced Hodgkin's disease with chemotherapy: Long-term follow up of MOPP treated patients at NCI. Ann Int Med 92(5): 587.

DeVita VT, Henney JE, and Weiss RB (1980). Advances in the multimodal primary management of cancer. In: Stollerman, GH, (ed) "Advances in Internal Medicine," Vol 26. Memphis, Year Book Medical Publishers, p 115.

DeVita VT, Henney JE, Hubbard SM (1981). Estimation of numerical and economic impact of chemotherapy in the treatment of cancer. Proceedings of the 1980 International Symposium on Cancer. In: Burchenal JH, Oettgen HS, (eds.) "Cancer Achievements and Prospects for the 1980s," New York, Grune & Stratton, p 859.

DeVita VT, Fisher RI and Young RC (1977). Treatment of diffuse histiocytic lymphomas: New opportunities for the future. In: Staquet MJ, and Tagnon HJ, (eds) "Recent Advances in Cancer Treatment," New York: Raven Press, p 39.

DeVita VT (1981). Recent perspectives on the development of drug resistance and some more good news. In: Salmon SE, Jones SE, (eds) "Adjuvant Therapy of Cancer," III. New York: Grune & Stratton, p 3.

DeVita VT Jr (1982). Hodgkin's disease: Conference summary and future directions. Cancer Treat Rep 66(4):1045.

DeVita VT (1982). Principles of chemotherapy. In: DeVita VT, Helman S, Rosenberg SA, (eds) "Cancer: Principles and Practices of Oncology," New York: Lippincott, p 379.

Fisher B, Slack NM, Bross IDJ (1969). Cancer of the breast: size of neoplasm and prognosis. Cancer 24:1071.

Fisher RI, DeVita, VT, Hubbard SM, Jaffe ES, Cossman J, Wesley R, Chabner, BA, and Young RC (1982). Improved survival of diffuse aggressive lymphomas following treatment with ProMACE-MOPP chemotherapy. Abstract C-627, ASCO Abstracts 161.

Frei E III, Jaffe AN, Gero M. et al (1978). Guest editorial: Adjuvant chemotherapy of osteogenic sarcoma: Progress and perspectives. J Natl Cancer Inst 60(1):3.

Furth J, Kahn MC (1937). The transmission of leukemia of mice with a single cell. Am J Cancer 31:276.

Goldie JH, Coldman AJ, Gudauskas GA (1982). Rationale for the use of alternating non-cross-resistant chemotherapy. Cancer Treatment Rep 66(3):439.

Goldie JH, Coldman AJ (1979). A mathematical model for relating the drug sensitivity of tumors to their spontaneous mutation rate. Cancer Treatment Rep 63(11-12):1727.

Gunduz N, Fisher B, Saffer EA (1979). Effective surgical removal on the growth and kinetics of residual tumor. Cancer Res 39:3861.

Hanson H, Koziner B, Clarkson B (1981). Marker and kinetic studies in non-Hodgkin's lymphomas. Am J Med 71:107.

Heppner GH, Dexter DL, DeNucci T, Miller FR, Calabresi P (1978). Heterogeneity in tumor sensitivity among tumor cell subpopulations of a single mammary tumor. Cancer Res 38(11, Pt.1): 3758.

Hubbard SM, Chabner BA, DeVita VT, Simon R, Berard CW, Jones RB, Garvin AJ, Canellos GP, Osborne GK, Young RC. (1982) Histologic progression in non-Hodgkin's lymphoma. Blood 59(2): 258.

Hutchison DJ and Schmid FA (1973). Cross-resistance and collateral sensitivity. In: Mihich E (ed) "Drug Resistance and Selectivity: Biochemical and Cellular Basis," New York: Academic Press, p 73.

Law LW (1952). Origins of the resistance of leukemic cells to folic acid antagonists. Nature 169: 628.

Ling V (1975) Drug resistance and membrane alteration in mutants of mammalian cells. Can J Genet Cytol 17:503.

Ling V (1978). Genetic aspects of drug resistance in somatic cells. In: Schabel FM, (ed) "Antibiotics and chemotherapy," Basel: S Karger, p 191.

Ling V (1982). Genetic basis of drug resistance in mammalian cells. In: Bruchovsky N, Goldie JH (eds) "Drug and Hormone Resistance in Neoplasia," Florida: CRC Press, (in press).

Longo DL, Young RC, DeVita VT (1982). What is so good about the "good prognosis" lymphoma. In: Williams CJ, Whitehouse M, (eds) "Recent Advances in Clinical Oncology," Edinburgh: Churchill Livingstone, p 223.

Luria SE, Delbruck M. (1943). Mutations of bacteria from virus sensitivity to virus resistance. Genetics 28:491.

Martin DS (1981). The scientific basis for adjuvant chemotherapy. Cancer Treatment Rev 8:169.

Mendelsohn, ML (1962). Autoradiographic analysis of cell proliferation in spontaneous breast cancer in C3H mouse. III. The growth fraction. J Natl Cancer Inst 28:1015.

Salles B, Charcosset Y-V, Jacquemin-Sablon A (1982). Isolation and properties of Chinese hamster lung cells resistant to ellipticine derivatives. Cancer Treatment Rep 66(2):327.

Salmon SE (1977). Kinetic rationale for adjuvant chemotherapy for cancer. In: Salmon SE, Jones SE, (eds) "Adjuvant Therapy of Cancer," Amsterdam, North Holland: Elsevier/North Holland Biomedical Press.

Santoro A, Bonnadonna G, Veronesi U (1978). Patterns of relapse and survival in operated breast cancer with positive and negative axillary nodes. Tumori 64:241.

Santoro A, Bonnadonna G, Bonfante V, and Valagussa P (1982). Alternating drug combinations in the treatment of advanced Hodgkin's disease. N Engl J Med 306:770.

Schabel FM (1975). Concepts for systemic treatment of micrometases. Cancer 35:15.

Schimke RT, Kaufman RJ, Alt FW, Kellems RF (1978). Gene amplification and drug resistance in cultured murine cells. Science 202:1051.

Simonovitch L (1976). On the nature of hereditable variation in cultured somatic cells. Cell 7:1.

Simpson- Herren L, Sanford AH, Holmquist JP (1976). Effects of surgery on the cell kinetics of residual tumor. Cancer Treatment Rep 60:1749.

Simpson-Herren L, Springer TA, Sanford AH, Holmquist JP (1977). Kinetics of metastases in experimental tumors. In: Day SP, Meyers WPL, Stanley P, Garattini S, Lewis MG, (eds) "Cancer Invasion and Metastases: Biologic Mechanisms in Therapy," New York: Raven Press, p 117.

Skipper HE (1978). Cancer Chemotherapy I. Reasons for success and failure of treatment of murine leukemias with the drugs now employed in treating human leukemias. Ann Arbor, University Microfilms International.

Skipper HE, Schabel FM Jr, and Wilcox WS (1964). Experimental evaluation of potential anti-cancer agents XII. On the criteria and kinetics associated with "curability" of experimental leukemia. Cancer Chemotherapy Rep 35:1.

Steel GG (1979). The utility of cell kinetic data in the design of therapeutic schedules. (editorial). Int J Radiat Oncol Biol Phys 5(1):145.

Steel GG, Stephens TC (1979). The relation of cell kinetics to cancer chemotherapy. Adv Pharmacol Chemother 10:137.

Tannock I (1978). Cell kinetics and chemotherapy: a critical review. Cancer Treatment Rep 62(8): 1117.

Weiss RB, DeVita VT (1979). The dilemma regarding postoperative chemotherapy in primary carcinoma of the colon. Surg Gynecol Obstet 149(2):267.

Weiss RB, DeVita VT (1979). Multimodal primary cancer treatment (adjuvant chemotherapy): Current results and future prospects. Ann Int Med 91(2):251.

Weiss RB, Henney JE, DeVita VT (1981). Multimodal treatment of primary breast carcinoma: Analysis of accomplishments and problem areas. Amer J Med 70:844.

Yankee RA, DeVita VT, Perry S (1968). The cell cycle of leukemia L1210 cells in vivo. Cancer Res 27(1):97.

Young RC, DeVita VT, Perry S (1969). The thymidine ^{14}C and ^{3}H double-labeling technique in the study of the cell cycle of L1210 leukemia ascites tumor in vivo. Cancer Res 29:1581.

13th International Cancer Congress, Part A
Current Perspectives in Cancer, pages 71–105
© 1983 Alan R. Liss, Inc., 150 Fifth Avenue, New York, NY 10011

CANCER EPIDEMIOLOGY: PAST, PRESENT AND FUTURE

C.S. Muir

International Agency for Research on Cancer

150, Cours Albert Thomas, Lyon, France

Cancer epidemiology in 1982 is well established as a discipline, no longer considered as a curiosity of marginal interest, far removed from the reality of the diagnosis and treatment of the cancer patient and from the basic laboratory and animal research which many believed would yield, not only the cause and mechanisms, but perhaps also the hitherto elusive cure for cancer. The cancer epidemiologist is regarded today as pares inter paribus.

In this review I shall briefly examine the events which have lead to the emergence of epidemiology as a discipline of critical importance, examine several aspects of the situation today and then address the problems, scientific and other, that are likely to preoccupy, vex and excite cancer epidemiologists over the next ten years.

Place of Epidemiology in Carcinogenesis

Before beginning I would like to place epidemiology in perspective. My rather simple concept of carcinogenesis is given in the Figure below:

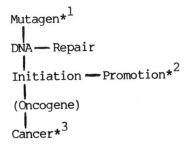

Mutagen*[1]
|
DNA — Repair
|
Initiation — Promotion*[2]
|
(Oncogene)
|
Cancer*[3]

In such a model the epidemiologist operates at the points marked by an asterisk*, seeking at *1 and *2 to identify exposures in the cancer patient *3 associated with an increased risk, exposures which he may or may not be able to characterise as either due to mutagenesis or promotion. Location *3 also represents the collection of descriptive data on the frequency and distribution of the disease.

THE PAST

Cancer epidemiology, as we know it today, probably began in 1950. The publication of the report on the Oxford Symposium on the Geographical Pathology and Demography of Cancer, organized by the Council for the Coordination of International Congresses of Medical Sciences under the auspices of the World Health Organization and the United Nations Educational, Scientific and Cultural Organization, summarized much of the available knowledge, drew attention to the importance of a multidisciplinary approach and emphasized the cardinal importance of lifestyle factors in the causation of many common cancers (Clemmesen, 1950).

True, there had been epidemiological life before 1950, the highlights being admirably reviewed by Clemmesen (1965) in the first volume of his series Statistical Studies in Malignant Neoplasms. Much of the early observational work and speculation concerning oral cancer in India from 1910 onwards led to Orr's publication in 1933 clearly showing the link with betel quid chewing. The long controversy concerning the role of tobacco in lung cancer was resolved in 1940 with the publication by Muller of a case-control study from Cologne showing an eight-fold increased risk among smokers compared to non-smokers.

Despite this, and the insight shown by Sir Ernest Kennaway (1944) (who was primarily interested in chemical carcinogenesis) into the significance of the results of migrant studies, it is probably true that cancer epidemiology became news in 1950 with the publication of large studies on the association between lung cancer and smoking by Doll and Hill (1950) and Wynder and Graham (1950). These studies were preceded, and followed, by others looking at industrial risk - the carcinogenicity of asbestos, chromates, and beta-naphthylamine were soundly established. It became accepted that there were discrete carcinogens in the environment which caused cancer and whose removal, it was presumed, would result in a lowering of risk. Cancer was in other words preventable.

A parallel course can be traced for carcinogenic risk factors. Rigoni Stern (1844) confirmed the observation of Ramazzini (1700) on the differing risk for breast and uterus cancer in nuns compared to other women, just as Pott (1775) had drawn attention to the dangers of occupational exposure to soot. Janet Lane-Claypon published a case-control study of cancer of the breast and "associated antecedent conditions" such as age at marriage in 1928. A later series of studies by MacMahon et al. (1970), Rotkin and Cameron (1968) and others established a link between such aspects of life-style as age at the first full-term pregnancy and age at first sexual intercourse for cancers of the breast and cervix uteri respectively.

Following such investigations we begin to see the chronic disease epidemiologist use, as his homologues in the field of infectious disease had done for many years, the laboratory, to look at hormonal levels, evidence of viral infection, etc., in humans. This trend has continued. The probable elucidation of the causes of primary hepatocellular carcinoma, which in terms of numbers of persons affected world wide may be the commonest of all internal cancers, has resulted from a collaboration between epidemiologists, chemists and mycologists (aflatoxin) and immunologists and virologists (hepatitis B virus). Indeed, for this cancer a trial of the effect of a vaccine against hepatitis B virus is now eminently feasible. There are, of course, other good reasons for deploying the hepatitis B vaccine than primary cancer of the liver. Although vaccines for breast cancer had been mooted, these were never developed as for this cancer the viral hypothesis was not sustained. Nonetheless epidemiologists had given thought to their evaluation (Higginson et al., 1971).

In 1980, MacMahon considered that in the previous decade the major advances in epidemiology had been in the development of an appropriate methodology unique to the field and in the substantial increase in the incorporation of biochemical, immunological and other laboratory evaluations into epidemiological studies and, indeed, epidemiological thinking. For three major cancers, primary liver cell cancer, breast cancer and large bowel cancer, he considered that the barriers to solution were now logistic rather than conceptual.

In all these studies descriptive epidemiologists have played their role, the gradual unravelling of cancer patterns over the years leading to the formulation of hypotheses later tested by their colleagues in analytical epidemiology. The UICC Committee on Geographical Pathology and its subcommittee on Africa, stimulated not only description, but analysis: that on Cancer Incidence was responsible for the first two volumes of "Cancer Incidence in Five Continents".

The foregoing has sketched the framework in which cancer epidemiology has developed. Its extension has been very patchy and there are still sizeable portions of both developed and developing worlds where cancer epidemiology is, to be charitable, rudimentary, although there are indications that this may change within the next 25 years.

EPIDEMIOLOGY TODAY

MacMahon and Pugh (1970) defined epidemiology as "use of knowledge on the frequency and distribution of disease in the search for determinants." Descriptive epidemiologists ascertain and describe the frequency: analytical epidemiologists tend to look for the exposures responsible. The two disciplines are complementary and overlap.

Descriptive Epidemiology

Cancer Registration

Cancer Incidence data are becoming more widely available. The most recent issue of "Cancer Incidence in Five Continents" (Waterhouse et al., 1982) contains data from 103 populations in 79 registries from 32 countries. Many of these registries have not been in existence for long enough to do much more than provide incidence data: their potential value as a source of end-points for cohort studies has still to be realized. While the reliability of numerators (the number of cases) improves, it is currently the denominators (the populations at risk) which give rise to concern in the shape of changing boundaries and underestimation of segments of a population.

It has recently become fashionable to try to establish cancer registries, often at a national level, on the grounds that these "are a good thing" and "might be useful" irrespective of other needs and priorities. Cancer registries have their place but their creation, extent of coverage and utilization, particularly in developing countries, need to be reviewed realistically. Nonetheless there is a great need for such registries in selected regions of Africa, Asia and Latin America.

Maps

Descriptive epidemiologists have re-discovered the map. The first cancer atlas – for England and Wales – dates back to 1875 (Haviland). Following publication of cancer mortality patterns in England and Wales in 1960 by Howe and the NCI county mortality atlas (Mason et al., 1976), a large number of similar atlases have appeared. Possibly the most interesting and best produced of these is the Cancer Mortality Atlas for China (1981): perhaps the most informative is that for the Netherlands (1980) presenting data for 40 areas within the country with a wealth of supporting information. It is when one tries to compare atlases, particularly for neighbouring countries, that problems such as size of area, standard population used, etc. arise. IARC is currently trying to produce a cancer mortality atlas presenting data in a uniform manner for Western Europe.

The exploitation of the different cancer patterns observed in the cancer atlases has however been tardy. Fraumeni, Blot, Hoover and others have pursued several of the interesting features of the US county maps. In New Jersey an extensive analysis has been undertaken within the state. In Japan, Ohno and Aoki (1977) have looked for clustering of bladder cancer.

The data used for the production of maps have also been used for correlation exercises but in such analyses the spatial aggregations or auto-correlations frequently ob-

served on the maps are lost or ignored and erroneous conclusions may be reached. The cartographic epidemiologist has
still much to learn from geographers and demographers if he
is to derive the maximum from his data.

Relative Frequency

IARC is currently trying to obtain relative frequency
information from many parts of the globe in an attempt to
build up the map of world cancer patterns and to use this to
derive hypotheses. In this respect the efforts of Brazilian
pathologists are of the greatest interest (Torloni and
Brumini, 1978). Their forthcoming publication giving the
distribution of some 370 000 cancers by age, sex and site,
according to the ICD-O, by province and district will provide an excellent feeling for the distribution of microscopically diagnosed cancers in that vast country. In
Algeria, Yaker and Dekkar (1980) have carried this one step
further, calculating minimum incidence rates relating the
microscopically diagnosed cancers to a census population.
While relative frequency data of this nature are clearly
biased, it is of interest that the cancer patterns uncovered
by the atlas of China reflect to a remarkable degree those
appearing in previous series of relative frequency figures
(Hu and Yang, 1959) lung cancer being possibly the only site
to have changed substantially over the years.

Time Trends

Time-trends have been recently studied in some detail
(Magnus, 1982) and there has been renewed interest in
birth-cohort analyses and in descriptive epidemiology in
general.

Standardization

For the presentation of incidence and mortality data
more and more material is published standardized to the
"world" standard population first proposed by the late
Professor Segi (as well as in several countries to a
national standard age-distribution). Increasing use is made
of the cumulative rate, a close approximation to the lifetime risk of contracting, or dying from, a specified cancer
in the absence of other causes of death (Day, 1976).

The past four years have seen the introduction of the 9th Revision of the ICD (International Classification of Diseases), the cancer section of which is wholly compatible with the ICD-O (WHO, 1976) and SNOMED (Standardized Nomenclature of Medicine). The importance of these tools, now cross-referenced to the International Histopathological Classification of Tumours of WHO, the so-called "Blue books", cannot be over-emphasized in that their increasing utilisation in many parts of the world helps to standardise diagnostic terms, and brings together the classifications, such as ICD, used by health administrators and those used by diagnostic histopathologists who confirm the presence of, and give a label to, over 80% of cancers.

The International Association of Cancer Registries continues to probe such matters as coding practices and the handling of multiple primaries in an effort to improve international comparability. From Canada, Last and his colleagues have embarked on a dictionary of epidemiological terms sponsored by the International Epidemiological Association.

Analytical Epidemiology

Current work in analytical epidemiology will not be systematically reviewed but much of what is underway is discussed in the following text which is largely based on a consideration of priorities and their implications.

PRIORITY

There are few epidemiologists and, as epidemiological studies take a long time to conduct and analyse, it is of some importance that effort be concentrated on the more important problems.

Occupation

At the time of the 12th International Cancer Congress the epidemiological world was abuzz with a claim that up to 20-40% of human cancers were related to occupational exposures. These claims, which never appeared in the refereed medical literature, would, if correct, have implied a massive investment in industrial studies, probably to the exclusion of. other forms of epidemiological enquiry. All the more so as it had been suggested that several exposures, such as asbestos, would result very shortly in a cancer epidemic. This report lead to a great deal of public anxiety, questionable advice was given to those exposed to asbestos, and there was considerable pressure on various branches of governmental and health services and on epidemiologists to tackle this problem (see Peto and Schneiderman, 1981).

The OPCS (Office of Population Censuses and Surveys, 1978) report on occupational mortality in England and Wales 1970-1972 is of the greatest significance in that it suggested that, in these countries at least, nearly 90% of the differences in cancer risk between occupational groups was likely to stem from the lifestyle habits of the social class from which a given occupation is drawn rather than from the exposures at work per se (Fox and Adelstein, 1978)

Other assessments of the relative importance of at-work exposures were remarkably consistent (Wynder and Gori, 1977, Higginson and Muir, 1979, Doll and Peto, 1981), lying in the 2-5% range. There is, however, no room for complacency. Cancers due to at-work exposures are preventable and the public has the right to demand a safe product from a safe workplace.

The number of persons exposed to a suspect industrial carcinogen in any one plant or indeed country may be quite small and hence it may be difficult to accumulate sufficient numbers of persons to assess risk. According to McMichael (1981) the dominant impression of studies of occupational risk is of people "working in a lamentably piecemeal fashion, doing little studies dotted all over the place with no adequate standardization of measurements and no good ability to pool data or to make satisfactory conclusions". The need is for "some central work, properly coordinated and widely supported". Indeed the type of coordination that IARC can provide and has provided in the field of manufacture of man-made mineral fibres (Saracci et al., 1982). (see Parochialism below).

Lifestyle Cancer

A broad consensus would now appear to have been reached on the relative importance of the major categories of cancer causation. Independent estimates by Wynder and Gori (1977) in the US, Higginson and Muir (1979) for UK and India, and more recently by Doll and Peto (1981), again for the US, are remarkably consistent in suggesting that one-third of cancers in men and perhaps two-thirds in women are due to lifestyle factors other than tobacco and alcohol consumption.

Yet, it is here that the epidemiologist feels himself at sea. True, he has shown in many parts of the world that age at first pregnancy influences risk for breast cancer, that age of first sexual intercourse and promiscuity are linked with cancer of the cervix uteri, that sunlight exposure increases malignant melanoma risk, that there is a fair chance that consumption of fresh fruit and vegetables protects against gastric cancer and that the same is true for dietary fibre and large bowel cancer, but he has little idea how many of these factors operate. With a view to possible rational prevention the main thrust of effort must thus be to dissect out how diet and other aspects of life-style influence the all too common cancers of the digestive and genital tracts.

If lifestyle is so important, why are there so few attempts being made to study it in some depth. I believe it is because we still do not have sufficient knowledge of the physiology of the human body and of its reactions to diet, pregnancy and the like. The needed progress will not occur in a vacuum; it is the epidemiologist who has to show where he needs help. It was the dietary fibre theory of Burkitt and Cleave that led epidemiologists to assess the influence of this part of diet on cancer risk. In so doing the laboratory collaborators rapidly discovered the inadequacies of traditional concepts on the composition of faeces and the nature and role of fibre, devising new analytical techniques and separating fibre into a series of non-starch poly-saccharides (Englyst et al., 1982).

Our perception of cancer causation is governed by the concept of attack of the DNA by mutagens resulting in transformed or initiated cells whose progression to malignancy may be enhanced by promoting agencts or arrested by inhibitors (see Figure). Such agents are usually seen as originating outside the body. It is recognised, however, that some (e.g. nitrosamines) can be formed in the stomach from apparently innocuous dietary precursors (e.g. nitrate and secondary amines). Bile acids, believed to act as promoters, are essentially endogenous as are the steroid hormones. It is in this area the epidemiologist needs help.

Study of Diet and Cancer

Many hold (unlike Graham and Mettlin, 1979) that retrospective enquiry into past dietary habits is of little value and pin their hopes on the prospective cohort study.

Hirayama (1981a), who has now followed a quarter of a million Japanese for 15 years, asked collaborating subjects a relatively narrow range of questions. Many of these questions on intake and frequency of intake of foodstuffs have yielded results on the protective effect of green/yellow vegetables in smokers, the influence of milk and milk products on gastric cancer and of meat on cancer of the pancreas, results which can be tested in other circumstances by a case–control approach.

Can we improve on Hirayama's techniques for the cohorts to be assembled in the next few years? Are the methods for assessing diet any better than they were 15 years ago? Given the considerable variation in diet over seasons, and perhaps over time, would it make sense to examine diet as such, or rather indirect markers in say faeces and blood? If so, how frequently should these specimens be collected? The various other aspects of lifestyle such as cigarette and alcohol consumption could be monitored by annual questionnaires. If the output of urinary mutagens is shown to be of significance, how frequently could these be determined by, say, a test–tape approach? Would it be worth monitoring the output of, say, N-nitrosoproline to assess the amount of endogenous nitrosation. The methods currently available for this estimation (Oshima and Bartsch, 1981) are fairly complex. One could also ask if endogenous nitrosation is significant. Should dietary mutagens such as occur in onions (Sugimura and Nagao, 1979) give cause for concern?

Do we know sufficient about these and other factors to plan the type of cohort study which would yield definitive results? Perhaps not, but if biological material and dietary homogenates are stored these can be examined, possibly on a case-control basis, as new methods and hypotheses emerge. The longer the delay in establishing the cohort - the longer it will take for the end-points to appear.

Carcinogens and Carcinogenic Factors

Higginson and Muir (1979) re-emphasized the critical distinction to be made between carcinogens and carcinogenic risk factors. In terms of prevention, avoidance of the former (tobacco, excess sunlight, excess alcohol, at-work exposures) can be guaranteed to result in a fall in risk. While the descriptive and analytical epidemiological evidence for the existence of carcinogenic risk factors such as age at first full term pregnancy is good, intervention may be difficult and yield unexpected and perhaps unwanted results. On the face of it measures to reduce the age at first pregnancy - thus reducing breast cancer risk - might increase the risk of cancer of the cervix uteri. The population of Karelia (Finland) which eats a high fibre diet has a low rate of large bowel cancer and very high mortality rates from ischaemic heart disease. It is not until the metabolic effect of the elements of the diet has been assessed - singly and in combination and including possible endogenous carcinogen formation - that it will be ethical to propose a "safer" diet.

Despite the current evidence it is possible that the protagonists of the lifestyle school, myself included, are wrong. Indeed, deep down I would like to be wrong, because there are many aspects of my present lifestyle that I enjoy. Demonstration by Ross and Bras (1965), following related studies by McCay et al. (1939), that the quantity of food eaten by an experimental animal may have a profound effect on longevity and on the incidence of spontaneous cancer, is disquieting.

Current Epidemiological Research

What are epidemiologists doing to-day? The answer is, more or less what their teachers did: perusal of the Directory of the Clearing-House for On-going Research in Cancer Epidemiology shows that there has been very little change in the sites of cancer studied between 1977 and 1981. Over these five years there has been an increase in use of the cohort study, largely in relation to industrial risk. As many such cohort studies are not evaluable as the smoking experience of cohort members is not known, the case-control study within the cohort is being increasingly attempted. The case-control study is still in the ascendent (Cole, 1979) but is subject to the limitations of memory bias and difficulties in exposure assessment. Several statisticians are trying to evaluate the degree of error that can be tolerated.

Studies on what one might describe as the "up and coming" cancers, prostate and pancreas, are very few. Lifestyle, although mentioned in many study abstracts, is investigated superficially and the existence of tumour promotion was mentioned but three times in 1,300 studies reported to the Clearing-House in 1981 (Muir and Wagner, 1981). There are remarkably few new hypotheses and many studies are copies of those conducted elsewhere or are devoted to dotting "i"s or crossing "t"s.

Medical research is not alone in playing it safe. The OECD (Organization for Economic Cooperation and Development) in a monograph discussing science and technology policy for the 1980's noted that for research and development expenditures "in the 1970's there has been a practically universal tendency in industry to turn from long-term research to short-term research entailing few risks".

Research funding

Cancer research funding was relatively liberal in the 1970's. I can only speculate on the reasons for lack of originality and timidity we now see. First, it could be that epidemiology does not attract original thinkers. Second, original or speculative thought is stifled by the peer review system. Horrabin (1982) suggests that research funds should be allocated by "lay" committees comprised of persons experienced in some other field who might be more able to see the wood than the trees. Has the influx of research funds in the form of grants in the long term been detrimental due to demands for quick results and elimination of projects based on a hunch or speculation?

Quick results cannot be expected from a forward cohort study - 10 years is a reasonable minimum time. Who would fund Hirayama's cohort, the Framingham study or the Busselton study to-day? Is it significant that it is a private body - the American Cancer Society - that will contribute substantially to the next large cohort study in United States?

How much of a scientist's time is devoted to writing or reviewing grant applications? How often do the rules change? How often does reorganisation take place? How many of those present have not been reorganised in the past 5 years? Let me quote Petronius "We trained hard, but it seemed that everytime we were beginning to form up into teams, we would be reorganized. I was to learn that we tend to meet any new situation by reorganizing, and a wonderful method it can be for creating the illusion of progress while producing confusion, inefficiency, and demoralization". Petronius was writing in AD 66.

THE FUTURE

In recent years, according to Doll (1979), epidemiology has contributed to knowledge of cancer in five ways:

1. by demonstrating geographical and temporal variation in cancer,
2. by correlating incidence in different communities with the prevalence of social habits and environmental agents,
3. by comparing the experience of individuals with and without cancer,
4. by intervening to remove suspected agents and observing the results and
5. by making quantitative observations that test the applicability to man of models of the mechanism by which the disease is produced.

Doll stressed that joint investigation of dietetic factors by epidemiologists and laboratory workers offers the brightest prospect of discovering new ways of preventing cancer in the near future. Even the least perceptive will have gathered that I too plead for greater collaboration between epidemiologists and laboratory workers. The question is on which topics are we to join effort ?

The basic research world is in effervescence! Molecular biology, DNA adducts to chemical carcinogens, molecular genetics, the oncogene, promotion, mutagens and promutagens - surely here there must be new tools for the epidemiologist to apply in conjunction with his laboratory counterpart. Yet, while it is exciting for the laboratory scientist to devise new techniques and new methods - their routine application is frequently another matter (serum is usually more welcome than faeces!). To analyse 20 samples is a pleasure; over a hundred becomes intolerable drudgery unless the method can be automated. But it is likely that for many studies much larger numbers would be needed and recourse to routine or commercial laboratories, with all the problems that this may entail, will be needed.

Promotion

The study of promotion would seem worth intensive effort. Berenblum (1980), speaking on cancer prevention as a realisable goal, stated that the primary rapid initiating phase of carcinogenesis is now generally accepted as being brought about by gene mutation, providing the cell with new tumour-type information and converting it into a potential or dormant tumour cell. He suggested that once the enzymes responsible for repair are identified it might be possible to stimulate their action and encourage the repair, thereby blocking any further carcinogenic action. (Cairns (1981) seems to suggest that mutagens attacking "natural" DNA sequences may be of lesser importance than those affecting transposed segments). This area of activity is clearly not epidemiological although the evaluation of the effects of such intervention would be.

Berenblum went on to state "interference with the promoting phase of carcinogenesis would seem to offer the best prospects for cancer prevention, if only because the promoting phase covers most of the latent period of carcinogenesis (which, in humans, may be 30 years or more)...". Describing several examples involving interference with the promoting phase, discovered by trial and error, he noted how much more logical it would be to discover how promoting action operates and then design specific methods of blocking the process, believing that we seemed to be getting closer and closer to doing this. Berenblum implied that a general preventive measure is possible. I would suggest that we may have to proceed on a promoter by promoter basis.

Identification of Promoters

To the epidemiologist a promoter is not essentially different from an initiator, since neither bears an identifying label. Both are likely to be present in some portion of the external or internal environment. Their existence can sometimes by inferred from examination of age-incidence curves, the behaviour of risk on withdrawal of a promotor-containing agent (Day, 1982) or on the existence of a form of cancer - as in the prostate - which apparently does not progress without further stimulation (Breslow et al., 1977). Can the laboratory scientist help us by identifying promotors? As noted above in the section on lifestyle and diet the process is in the nature of a feedback loop with the epidemiologist drawing attention to areas for investigation and vice versa.

Susceptibility

When one reflects on the epidemiological method, how crude it seems. Essentially we behave as if human beings were identical in all respects other than exposures to a few agents. Yet we have overwhelming evidence that genetically we are anything but similar. How can such diversity be taken into account? Put in another way how important is genetic susceptibility? The hunt for cancer families, the gastric cancer/blood group A relationship, the DNA repair defects in patients with Xeroderma pigmentosum, and the discovery of

HLA/cancer associations have by and large not really improved our ability to identify either high risk groups nor indicated how susceptibility operates, nor how to advise most such persons on how to reduce risk.

In a very elegant study in Iceland (Tulinius et al., 1982), the familial risk of breast cancer has been examined for the total population, revealing a 2.6 fold increase in risk for sisters and mothers of the breast cancer patients. As this cancer has increased in incidence in Iceland over the past 60 years, does this represent an increased frequency of a cancer susceptibility gene (very unlikely) or a rise in the "causes"? Here is surely an area for intensive multidisciplinary research.

Chemoprevention

Trials of Vitamin C, alpha-tocopherol and Vitamin A like substances as chemopreventive agents may now be justified. Their evaluation will require most careful monitoring of subjects over a long period of time.

BARRIERS TO PROGRESS

The epidemiologist comes up against many barriers. Some of these are natural - others erected by man. Several which appear important are discussed below.

Perception of Epidemiological Evidence

Epidemiology is an observational science and as such it is held by many to be of lesser value than the experimental approach in that a causal relationship is not easily established. In a sense we have to guess from our observations what the experiment was that produced the observed results.

Many fail to appreciate that a science based on probability means just that. The existence of an apparently healthy relative or friend who works in an asbestos mine, smokes 40 cigarettes a day and drinks a bottle of whisky each evening is quite compatible with each of these exposures being carcinogenic, a point frequently difficult to get across.

One of the criticisms levelled at the epidemiological approach is that industrial (and other) risks are discovered when it is too late – an increased risk, it is held, should be detected during the induction period. Epidemiology is not predictive. It can only assess the effects of exposures that have taken place and even here there are problems. While high risk groups may be identified, it is the chemists, immunologists and molecular biologists who are going to provide the tools to identify individuals likely to be at increased risk before cancers appear (Legator, 1981).

Parochialism

Risk differentials within a country are generally low. If a country is sufficiently large or multiracial, then there may be contrasting levels. International variations are frequently much larger, yet are but little exploited. The table below examines incidence for six populations in four countries (Denmark, Finland, Hawaii and New Zealand) for sites which have been in some way linked to intake of fat and dietary fibre. All these populations could be said to have access to good health services. Not only are the risk gradients substantial but the patterns of site vary, differences which any causal hypothesis must explain. Why the low level of large bowel cancer in Hawaiians and Maoris compared to Caucasian populations in the same country?

COMPARATIVE CANCER RISK FOR SELECTED CANCER SITES AND
POPULATIONS AROUND 1970[1]

	Females			Males	
	Breast	Corpus	Large Bowel	Large Bowel	Prostate
Caucasians*	++++	+++	++++	++++	+++
Hawaiians*	+++	+++	++	++	+
Maoris**	++	+++	+	+	+++
Non-maoris**	++	++	++++	++++	++
Danes	++	+	+++	+++	+
Finns	+	+	+	+	+
High/low***	80/22	32/10	35/14	38/12	42/20

*Resident in Hawaii
**Resident in New Zealand
***Rates age-adjusted to the "world" population standard,
derived from Waterhouse et al (1976) Prostate in Hawaiians
excepted, these patterns are largely preserved in more recent
data (Waterhouse et al., 1982) but differentials tend to be
smaller.

Who is going to coordinate such multinational investigations? I would suggest this is the role of IARC: Our
ability to do so is exemplified in international studies of
large bowel cancer (IARC Intestinal Micro-ecology Group,
1977; Jensen et al., 1982) and Man-Made Mineral Fibres
(Saracci et al., 1982). We clearly cannot undertake the
field work ourselves but coordination requires funds. The
amount available for mounting epidemiological studies from
IARC is but $500,000 a year. What could we not do with 10
times that amount?

Identification of Migrants

The world is full of migrant populations. Yet little
has been done to exploit their differences in cancer risk
from those of the countries of origin and settlement
(Haenszel being a notable exception). The United Kingdom has

now substantial populations of Caribbeans, Indians and Pakistanis. Study of their cancer patterns on arrival and the effect of length of stay, changes in diet, etc. are very difficult as the appropriate denominator information does not exist and ethnic appartenance is not given on death certificate or hospital record. The epidemiologist is thus in general faced by two problems - illegal migration (migrants figure in the numerator but not denominator) and government policy (migrants do not officially exist) - which prevent observation, let alone interpretation, of the results of great natural experiments in which populations move from one set of carcinogens and carcinogenic risk factors to another.

Access to the Tools of the Trade

Despite increasing awareness of the importance of epidemiology for the detection of risk, the past ten years have seen the advent of a powerful sclerosant or blocking agent in the shape of confidentiality. In none of the countries of Western Europe where access to the death certificate by name has been prohibited has there been any indication of a liberalisation of the rules, even under the most stringent restrictions. A cancer registry in the Federal Republic of Germany ceased operation for a year until the legal position of physicians reporting cases to the registry had been clarified. While mortality and incidence data continue to be published, there is an increasing reluctance to publish tables with less than 5 to 10 persons in a cell, lest an individual might be linked to a particular disease. Despite the abundance of environmental data collected routinely by many public bodies, this is frequently classified or presented in such a form as to be useless for correlation and hypothesis formulation.

The investigator wishing to conduct a case-control study has to clear an increasing number of hurdles in the shape of review and ethical committees, the viability of an investigation frequently being imperilled by one or two individuals who can in effect wield a veto. The cheapest and most effective method of linking at-work exposures to a health effect, namely, the cohort study, is made impossible by the refusal either to provide lists of those exposed or by destruction of records. Permission to link such lists to death certificate, cancer registry or other relevant records may be refused. Record destruction might be to save space or it could be to prevent subsequent study and possible claims for compensation. To avoid penalizing companies which do preserve and give access to records national and international efforts are needed to ensure that such documents are kept <u>by all</u> for 50 years.

IARC continues to press governments to limit the harmful effects of confidentiality on epidemiological research.

There are however still many countries where responsible epidemiological research is not only possible but encouraged and, when justified, matching of computer files is authorized. Despite the public's fear of "names in the computer" modern cryptographic techniques enable the coding of names in a practically unbreakable form. Nonetheless Rothman's (1981) apocalyptic vision of the rise and fall of epidemiology is unfortunately all too realistic for comfort and the time has come for the whole cancer research community to take the offensive. I would like to stress that this is a matter that affects us all. No man is an island: even the basic scientist is mortal and dies from the same diseases as others. It seems to me that many of those who campaign actively for yet further restrictions on confidentiality are the same as those who demand, and rightly so, that there be a carcinogen-free environment. They do not see, or do not wish to see, the contradiction of their standpoints.

Manpower

Despite the brave words in the introduction to this communication about the place of the epidemiologist in the firmament, the science is poorly established, and with few practitioners, in much of the world. Where there are reasonable numbers of epidemiologists, there is a danger of schism resulting in a profession divided into two groups: the medically qualified sound on biology and poor in statistics and the statistically qualified weak in biology. This argues strongly for the existence of a critical mass of epidemiologists drawn from both backgrounds if a unit is to be successful. Sound training courses at centres of academic excellence are now available; governments need to ensure that their graduates have reasonable career prospects.

Small Relative Risk, Small Dose and Negative Study

It would be quite out of place in a plenary lecture to go into the minutiae of epidemiological methods. There are however several questions which require urgent resolution, namely, the small relative risk, the small dose and the negative study.

There is no consensus as to the significance of small increases in relative risk. Are these to be considered seriously or regarded as part of our "normal" background? It is easy to fall into the relative risk trap – the 400-fold increase in the incidence of angiosarcoma of the liver in vinyl-chloride kettle cleaners compared to the general population is somehow much more clamant than a relative risk of 1.5 due to an exposure affecting half a nation – although the number of cancers resulting from exposure to the "weaker" carcinogen would be very much larger. A case-control study can uncover relative risks of three or more for an exposure affecting half of the population with less than 100 cases and the same number of controls. To achieve statistical significance for a relative risk of 1.5 under the same circumstances would require 440 cases. This clearly would make the study expensive and if, as would be desirable for such a level of relative risk, the study has to be re-peated in several areas to see whether a similar trend is observed, then the investment in time, manpower and money becomes very large. Among the issues requiring urgent clari-fication are the role of coffee in pancreas cancer and the extent of the risk from passive smoking.

It has become fashionable to dissect case-control studies into numerous strata, and re-analyse the data, a procedure which may result in finding a small group with a raised relative risk. Such repeated carving of the cake will undoubtedly result in the emergence by chance of groups with significantly raised risk. It is easy to understand the temptation to have a "positive" finding.

The small relative risk has some interesting and equally intractable bed mates. First of these is the small

dose of carcinogens. What is the significance of the
temporal increase in asbestos bodies found in the lungs of
some populations? Is the asbestos released into the air on
braking a significant risk factor? Atmospheric pollution
would seem to be carcinogenic only in smokers (Vena, 1982).
What happens at very low dose levels of radiation?

Are such low doses from several sources additive or
multiplicative (is antagonism ever considered?). From the
prevention point of view in many countries half the
radiation comes from natural sources and most of the rest
from diagnostic X-rays (Jablon and Bailar, 1980). In
practical terms it is in diagnostic use that most of the
reduction in radiation exposure can be made. There are,
however, benefits to diagnostic X-ray.

A proportion of the case-control studies reported over
recent years, could be considered as negative in that the
relative risk was not statistically significantly different
from unity at the 5% level (Some studies underway, notably
those on nasal cancer in persons exposed to formaldehyde,
would not have a 80% chance of detecting a ten-fold relative
risk because of the very small numbers involved). There is a
curious reluctance, notably in relation to occupational exposures, to accept negative results. Two main reasons for
doubting a negative result are advanced: one is trivial, to
wit, if only the study had been larger, significance would
have been achieved. While this will always be true if the
numbers become very large, the relative risk could remain
the same. The second, much more difficult to accomodate, is
the argument that if follow-up had been longer, the effect
might have been larger, and significant. This could well be
true, but in general the longer it takes for an effect to
appear, the less likely is the carcinogen to be significant.
Nonetheless, one must be cautious for although the first
tumour of the bladder took 5 years to appear in betanaphthy-
lamine distillers, after 30 years all eventually developed
this particularly horrible form of malignant disease. Such
individuals were, of course, exposed to very high levels of
the chemical.

Computers and Statistics

The analysis of many epidemiological studies would be virtually impossible without the aid of the computer. It is used to "clean" data about the individuals participating in a study, for reorganization of data. The ready division into numerous classes and strata, and the computation of various indices requiring iteration would be virtually impossible without this assistance. The existence of numerous package programmes free the investigator and the statistician from the hum-drum tasks of designing tabulations and computing simple indices. Nonetheless, such packages never tell the inexperienced investigator which of the many indices or techniques so readily available are appropriate for his data.

Despite its speed and capacity for storage, the computer of today still largely follows a Neumannian sequential way of processing. As long ago as 1798 Van Haller stated "In nature, varied phenomena are linked into a net-work rather than a chain, but man grasps only a chain of relationship because he cannot describe in words more than one relationship at a time". Will the 5th generation of computers help to overcome this?

The advent of the statistician has been a two-edged weapon. Good statisticians are rare. Statistical referreeing of papers on epidemiological and other topics in medical science is of unequal quality, an ethical as well as scientific issue (Altman, 1982). Failure to use confidence intervals, failure to state the magnitude of the effect that the study in question could detect, misuse of the p value and the correlation coefficient and indeed the whole theory of statistical tests are common.

Mathematical modelling for many aspects of cancer research periodically enjoys a renaissance. Many models are useful but the words of Nobel Prize winner Leontieff (1982), speaking of a parallel field, are worth bearing in mind. "Page after page of professional economic journals are filled with mathematical formulas leading the reader from sets of more or less plausible but entirely arbitrary assumptions to precisely stated but irrelevant conclusions".

THE EPIDEMIOLOGIST LOOKS AT THE CONTEMPORARY SCENE

Epidemiologists are at the cross-road that link clinicians, statisticians, computer specialists and experimentalists to the population in which the cancers occur. Epidemiologists are in a position to evaluate the results of the control measures that public health administrators and politicians may decide to implement. From this privileged Olympian position we should have a certain perspective on the cancer problem as a whole, biased it is true towards people and the world in which they live.

Progress and lack thereof

On the credit side of the ledger we have the truly fantastic progress made in many areas of experimental cancer research. Time will show how much of this has relevance to human disease: I believe that an increasing number of outstanding basic research scientists are increasingly conscious of the need to relate their work to that of the epidemiologists.

Written in red ink on the debit side is the depressing fact that for populations taken as a whole (not selected patient groups) the results of treatment for most common cancers have not really improved over the past 20 years (acute lymphatic leukaemia of childhood, choriocarcinoma and Hodgkin's disease are welcome exceptions).

The tobacco industry, checked but by no means conquered in a small number of developed countries, is energetically promoting its wares in the developing world. Here the cigarettes are frequently of the high tar and high nicotine varieties; nicotine fosters addiction. At a time when WHO is trying to curb tobacco use FAO (Food and Agriculture Organization of the United Nations) continues to advise such governments on tobacco planting and exploitation. In developed countries the current rises in female lung and possibly larynx cancer portend an epidemic.

One might have imagined that after so many years of study there was little more to discover about this addictive toxin. The finding by Hirayama (1981b) and Trichopoulos et al. (1981) that passive smoking by non-smokers carried a relative risk of over 2 for lung cancer may explain why some non-smokers develop the disease. Further studies are urgently needed for this may be a finding of major public health importance.

Screening for cancer of the cervix, carried out in many countries and which consumes a considerable amount of money and manpower, is only now being properly evaluated.

Informing the Public

The communication of the results of epidemiological studies to the public is an important issue. Inevitably the conclusions of some epidemiological studies will be wrong, the investigation may not be well designed, the choice of controls may be incorrect, or by chance an odd result may emerge.

The first report of a new risk is normally published in scientific journals accompanied by numerous reservations and caveats. This is often, and increasingly, accompanied by a press or television interview in which these entirely proper cautions are either thrown to the wind or omitted when the "break through" appears in print in the lay press. In consequence the public, continually deluged by such reports, and not being without common sense, in time comes to disregard them all. The overwhelming case against tobacco is weakened by each "scare" which is unwarranted.

At present there do not seem to be satisfactory mechanisms for providing the public with a reasonable assessment of the evidence. One possible approach would be to make greater use of that developed by IARC in the Monographs on the Evaluation of the Carcinogenic Risk of Chemicals to Humans. In preparing these monographs an international group of experts with specialized knowledge of the area meet for a week or more and thrash out a consensus opinion following evaluation of the published literature on mutagenicity tests, animal tests, and when available, the consequences of human exposures. While such evaluations may change over time as new evidence becomes available, they have the enormous benefit in that they represent a major degree of agreement on the part of experts selected from many portions of the world. In my opinion, these evaluations have to date been neither too conservative nor too bold.

While the IARC programme is moving from pure chemicals to include industrial processes, such as the rubber industry, other types of risk factor, such as those linked to diet or lifestyle, have not yet been evaluated.

Once an evaluation is made it is up to each country to interpret it in terms of its own legislative action. A body such as IARC cannot be aware of local circumstances and needs that must be taken into account in framing regulations.

Public attention is diverted from the major problems like tobacco by an increasing number of red herrings. Thus fluoridation of water is claimed to be the cause of cancer of unspecified sites. Scotland has recently seen a trial lasting 204 days, the longest ever, at a cost to public funds of over 3 million pounds to decide whether the Strathclyde Regional Council should cease to add fluoride "a horrible poison and a witches' brew" to water, this being the "technical" description put forward in the plaintiff's original submission.*

Antivivisectionists demonstrate outside medical laboratories against the use of animals for cancer research, carry out raids to free beagles used for smoking research, spray slogans on Sir Richard Doll's car. It is indeed ironical that Sir Richard, who has spent his professional life investigating humans, frequently the medical profession, should be singled out for such treatment. But if there have been demonstrations outside cigarette factories or automobile plants against these frequently lethal products I have yet to hear of them.

The wrong emphasis

Prevention remains a rather theoretical concept little applied other than to industrial risks or those risks perceived to be the responsibility of government such as food additives, pesticides, air and water pollution, radiation,

*Daily Telegraph, London, 28 July 1982

and the like. For these exposures in many countries an adversary position stultifies progress. Any preventive measure that implies or entails individual choice is frequently roundly rejected as infringing personal liberty.

I believe that if one were to send a questionnaire to a large number of people in any part of the developed world asking them to list the advances that they would most like to see in the next decade, "an end to war", "health for all" and "a cure for cancer", would be close to the head of this list. I would be willing to wager a large sum that "the prevention of cancer" would figure very rarely. Why this should be so is not clear. Most countries have the proverb: "Prevention is better than cure". Why not for cancer? I believe that this concept of cancer as a fire breathing dragon to be conquered by knights in shining armour rather than as a maggot to be stifled at birth distorts our priorities. Thomas Adams said it all in the 17th century:

"Hee is a better physician that keepes diseases off us, than hee that cures them being on us. Prevention is so much better than healing, because it saves the labour of being sick".

Yet, how much glory was attached to the conquest, by preventive measures, of smallpox?

It is fashionable to talk of risk-benefit assessments. These are not only difficult but rare. It is facile to say "whose risk?" and "whose benefit?". One only has to consider tobacco to realize how all-pervasive the "benefits" are and what immense financial dislocation a sudden total ban on this product would entail, an analysis which would stretch even Tinbergen. Should overnutrition be shown to be of great importance in digestive and genital tract cancer it will be interesting to see how governmental policies evolve particularly in those countries with large cereal and dairy product surpluses.

Perutz (1981) in an admirable unemotional, indeed, almost detached, article, examines the consequences of uncritical assessment of risk and benefit. "Finally it is becoming clear that the resources of science are limited and that we cannot expect it to give us greater agricultural productivity, more energy and better drugs indefinitely. We must learn to make the best use of what science has already provided and to accept a small measure of risk in return for its benefits. Our refusal to do so will place these benefits beyond the purse of the poorer inhabitants of the globe and ultimately, beyond the West".

While epidemiology is but one of the ways to find out more about our common foe, to the epidemiologist much of what is currently designated as cancer research seems highly academic, to be concerned mainly with mechanisms of carcino-genesis, and unlikely to yield information relevent to pre-vention. It is not always necessary to understand mecha-nisms to intervene effectively but for carcinogenic risk factors it may be prudent to acquire such understanding. While most of what is known about the factors that influence cancer risk is due to the epidemiologist, epidemiology is not the philosopher's stone. Epidemiology cannot transmute base metals (or false ideas) into gold (or the truth). It is, however, a touchstone which will ring true when hypo-theses are tested in man. An answer in man is still more valid for man than those derived from bacteria, mice or monkeys.

More research?

While it is customary to end lectures such as this with a call for further research and increased funding it is salutory to recall the words of two distinguished American scientists - Theobald Smith and O.W. Holmes. The former wrote: "Research cannot be forced too much; there is always the danger of too much foliage and too little fruit" : the latter : "A moment's insight is sometimes worth a lifetime's experience".

SYNTHESIS

Cancer epidemiology, as we know it today, probably began in 1950. Although there had been epidemiological life long before this time with descriptions of geographical patterns of cancer and the uncovering of both discrete car-cinogens and carcinogenic risk factors, it was the publica-tion that year of the large scale studies by Doll and Hill and Wynder and Graham, associating lung cancer with smoking, that attracted and stimulated scientific and public attention.

In recent years descriptive epidemiologists in their search for hypotheses have continued to assess world cancer patterns (although large gaps still exist in Africa, Asia and Latin America) and to improve data comparability by standardization of techniques, definitions and presentation. In an attempt to present cancer patterns as informatively as possible cancer maps are increasingly used. Time trends have enjoyed a resurgence of interest, particularly birth-cohort analyses. Analytical epidemiologists continue to uncover risk factors.

Descriptive and analytical evidence indicates that in many countries about one-third of cancers in males are due to tobacco and alcohol, one third to lifestyle factors (including diet) and about one in twenty to exposures at work. For females over half are likely to be associated with diet or lifestyle. The priorities for the next 10 years are thus clear - to determine how diet and other elements of lifestyle influence risk for the very common cancers of the digestive and genital tracts. It is obvious that solutions to this problem - which may first require further extensive investigation of physiological chemistry - can only come from the joint efforts of laboratory scientists and epidemiologists, a fact recognised over 30 years ago in the 1950 report on the Oxford Symposium on the Geographical Pathology and Demography of Cancer. The clarification of the causes of primary liver cancer exemplifies such collaboration between clinicians, chemists, mycologists, virologists, immunologists, etc. The identification of exogenous and endogenous promoters would currently seem to offer the best prospects for prevention, if only because this phase covers most of the induction period of human cancer.

For elucidation of the role of diet in cancer risk it is likely that large scale cohort studies lasting 10 to 15 years will be required; but the commitment to the long term funding needed for such cohort studies is far from assured.

The role of genetic susceptibility in breast and other common cancers has for too long been an enigma: this too is a priority area. In view of their prevalence, rapid answers are needed on the role of passive smoking and coffee drinking.

To achieve these ends there are numerous barriers to be overcome including confidentiality and other obstacles to record linkage, issues which increasingly hamper case-control and cohort studies and, ultimately, all progress in cancer prevention. The rapid and economical identification of cancer risk in persons exposed at work is only possible by the cohort study: it is ironical that those who press for confidentiality are often those who rightly demand a risk-free workplace. These are questions which ultimately affect all scientists – they are not only the problem of the epidemiologist. The small relative risk, the small dose and the negative study still pose problems of interpretation. There are too few epidemiologists and practical statisticians; the potential of the computer is not yet exploited.

At a time when countries are becoming increasingly homogeneous, parochialism results in the large international differences in cancer level being poorly exploited. As the numbers of persons exposed to a suspected industrial carcinogen may be small in any one country, pooling of data is essential. IARC has shown what can be done in these two domains.

Mechanisms for informing the public about cancer risk in a balanced manner need to be devised. The emphasis in our thinking needs to shift from cure to prevention. Yet, in many countries prevention is perceived to be the responsibility of government whose duty it is to protect the public against pollution of air, food, water and the workplace. Any measure that implies or entails personal choice is rejected as being an infringement to the liberty of the individual. Too much time is spent on questions of marginal importance and the development of control measures by adversary procedures stultifies progress.

How can the tobacco problem be resolved, and what will governmental policies be if overnutrition is shown to be a major risk factor for digestive and genital tract cancers? While intervention for discrete carcinogens such as asbestos can be guaranteed to eventually reduce risk the results of intervention for carcinogenic risk factors, unless their mechanisms are thoroughly understood, may be less predictable and entail other unwanted effects. Thus, on the face of it, a fall in the mean age of the first pregnancy would reduce breast cancer levels, but might also, by reducing the mean age at first coitus, increase the incidence of cervix uteri malignancy. Similar considerations apply to dietary intervention, notably in relation to heart disease and trials of chemopreventive agents may yet have unexpected side effects.

Yet, despite its imprecision, the problems of the long induction period and an inability to predict the effects of an exposure, epidemiology is the ultimate arbiter of risk for man. Most of what is known about the factors that influence cancer risk in humans is due to epidemiologists. To quote Charron (1601): "The true science and study of man is man!"

ACKNOWLEDGEMENTS

My colleagues were kind enough to review the text making many useful suggestions: Mrs A. Romanoff and Miss A.-M. Corre cheerfully typed the many versions.

Altman DG (1982) Statistics in medical journals, Statistics in Medicine 1:59.

Berenblum I (1980) Cancer prevention as a realizable goal. In Fortner JG, Rhoads JE (eds) "Accomplishments in Cancer Research 1980". General Motors Cancer Research Foundation. JB Lippincott Company, Philadelphia, Toronto. p 101.

Bras G, Ross MH (1965) Tumor incidence patterns and nutrition in the rat. J Nutr 87:245.

Breslow NE, Chan CW, Dhom G et al. (1977) Latent carcinoma of prostate at autopsy in seven areas. Int J Cancer 20:680.

Cairns J (1981) The origins of human cancer. Nature 289:353.

Centraal Bureau voor de Statistiek. (1980) "Atlas of Cancer Mortality in the Netherlands 1969-1978". Netherlands Central Bureau of Statistics, The Hague.

Chinese Institute of Medical Sciences (1981) "Atlas of Cancer Mortality in the People's Republic of China". Cancer Institute, Chinese Academy of Medical Sciences, China Cartographic Publishing House, Beijing, China.

Clemmesen J (ed) (1950) Symposium on Geographical Pathology and Demography of Cancer, Oxford, England. Paris: Council Int Org Med Sci.

Clemmesen J (1965) "Statistical Studies in Malignant Neoplasms. I Review and Results". Munksgaard, Copenhagen.

Cole P (1979) The evolving case-control study. J Chron Dis 32:15

Day NE (1976) A new measure of age-standardized incidence, the cumulative rate. In Waterhouse J et al (eds) "Cancer Incidence in Five Continents" Vol III. IARC Scientific Publications No 15. Lyon.

Day NE (1982) The epidemiological evidence of promoting effects. The example of breast cancer. In Hecker E et al (eds) "Carcinogenesis" Vol 7, New York, Raven Press.

Doll R (1979) The epidemiology of cancer. In: Fortner JG & Rhoads JE (eds) "Accomplishments in Cancer Research 1979". General Motors Cancer Research Foundation. JB Lippincott Company, Philadelphia, Toronto.

Doll R & Hill AB (1952) A study of the aetiology of carcinoma of the lung. Brit Med J 2:1271.

Doll R, Peto R (1981) The causes of cancer: Quantitative estimates of avoidable risks of cancer in the United States today. J Natl Cancer Inst 66:1191

Englyst H, Wiggins HS, Cummings JH (1982) Determination of the nonstarch polysaccharides in plant foods by gas-liquid chromatography of constituent sugars as alditol acetates. Analyst 107:307.

Fox AJ, Adelstein AM (1978) Occupational mortality: Work or way of life? J Epidemiol Community Health 32:73.

Graham S, Mettlin C (1979) Diet and colon cancer. Am J Epidemiol 109:1.

Haviland A (1875) The geographical distribution of diseases in Great Britain. London, Smith, Elder & Co.

Higginson J, de-The G, Geser A, Day NE (1971) An epidemiological analysis of cancer vaccines. Int J Cancer 7:565.

Higginson J, Muir CS (1979) Environmental carcinogenesis: Misconceptions and limitations to cancer control. J Natl Cancer Inst 63:1291.

Hirayama T (1981a) Proportion of cancer attributable to occupation obtained from a census, population-based, large cohort study in Japan. In Peto R and Schneiderman M. Loc. cit.

Horrobin D (1982) In praise of non-experts. New Scientist 94:842.

Howe M (1970) "National Atlas of Disease Mortality in the United Kingdom", Nelson, London.

Hu CH, Ch'in KY (1940) A statistical study of 2,179 tumors occurring in the Chinese. Chin Med J 58:381.

ICD-O (1976) (International Classification of Diseases for Oncology). World Health Organization, Geneva.

International Agency for Research on Cancer Intestinal Microecology Group (1977) Dietary fibre, transit time, faecal bacteria, steroids and colon cancer in two Scandinavian populations. Lancet ii:207.

Jablon S, Bailar JC III (1980) The contribution of ionizing radiation to cancer mortality in the United States. Prev med 9:219

Jensen OM, MacLennan R, Wahrendorf J (1982) Diet, bowel function, fecal characteristics, and large bowel cancer in Denmark and Finland. Nutr Cancer 4:5.

Kennaway EL (1944) Cancer of the liver in the Negro in Africa and America. Cancer Res 4:571.

Lane-Claypon EJ (1928) A further report on cancer of the breast with special reference to its associated antecedent conditions. Rep Min Health No 32, London.

Legator MS (1981) A realistic approach to monitoring high-risk populations by short-term procedures. In Peto R, Schneiderman MG loc cit p 355.

Leontief W (1982) Academic Economics. Science 217:104.

MacMahon B (1980) Cancer Epidemiology. In Fortner JG, Rhoads JE (eds). "Accomplishments in Cancer Research 1980." General Motors Cancer Research Foundation. JB Lippincott Company, Philadelphia, Toronto. p 235.

MacMahon B, Pugh TF (1970) "Epidemiology. Principles and Methods". Boston, Little Brown.

MacMahon B, Cole P, Lin T et al (1966) Age at first birth and breast cancer risk. Bull Wld Hlth Org 43:209.

Magnus K (1982) "Trends in Cancer Incidence", New York, Hemisphere.

Mason TJ, McKay FW, Hoover R, Fraumeni JF (1975) "Atlas of cancer mortality among US non-whites 1950-1969", US Govt Printing Office, Washington.

McCay CM, Maynard LA, Sperling G, Barnes LL (1939) Retarded growth, life span, ultimate body size and age changes in the albino rat after feeding diets restricted in calories. J Nutr 18:1.

McMichael AJ (1981) Needs for the future: A concluding discussion In Peto R and Schneiderman MG (eds) loc cit p 693.

Mueller FH (1940) Tabaksmisbrauch und Lebenkarzinom. Z Krebsforsch 49:57.

Muir CS, Wagner G (eds) (1981) "Directory of On-going Research in Cancer Epidemiology, 1981". IARC Scientific Publications No 38. Lyon, International Agency for Research on Cancer.

OECD (1981) Science and technology policy for 1980's. OECD, Paris.

Ohno Y, Aoki K (1977) Epidemiology of bladder cancer deaths in Japan. Gann 68:715.

OPCS (Office of Population Censuses and Surveys) (1978) Occupational mortality. The Registrar General's Decennial Supplement for England and Wales, 1970-1972. Series DS No 1. HMSO, London.

Orr IM (1933) Oral cancer in betel nut chewers in Travancore: Its aetiology, pathology, and treatment. Lancet 2:575.

Oshima H, Bartsch H (1981) Quantitative estimation of endogenous nitrosation in humans by monitoring N-nitrosoproline excreted in the urine. Cancer Res 41:3658.

Perutz M (1981) Why we need science. New Scientist 92:530.

Peto R, Schneiderman ME (1981) "Quantification of occupation and cancer". Banbury Report No 9. Cold Spring Harbor.

Pott P (1775) Chirurgical observations relative to the cataract, the polyps of the nose, the cancer of the scrotum, the different kinds of ruptures and the mortification of the toes and feet. London, Hawes, Clarke and Collins.

Ramazzini B (1700) De Morbis Artificum Diatriba, translation by WC Wright, Univ of Chicago Press, Chicago, 1940.

Rothman KJ (1981) Sounding boards. The rise and fall of epidemiology, 1950-2000 AD. N Engl J Med 304:600.

Rotkin ID, Cameron JR (1968) Clusters of variables influencing risk of cervical cancer. Cancer 21:4.

Saracci R, 14 collaborators (1982) Mortality and cancer incidence study of man-made mineral (vitreous) fibre production workers in seven European countries. Proceedings of Conference on Biological Effects of Man-made Mineral Fibres. WHO Copenhagen, 20-22 April 1982, (in press).

Stern Rigoni (1844) I Giornale per Servire al Progressi della Pathologia e della Terapeutica. 2:507, 1842. II Annali Universali di Medicina, 110:484, 1844.

Sugimura T, Nagao M (1979) Mutagenic factors in cooked foods. CRC Crit Rev Toxicol 6:189.

Torloni H, Brumini R (1978) Registro Nacional de Tumores. Rio de Janeiro, Ministry of Health.

Trichopoulos D, Kalandini A, Sparros L et al. (1981) Lung cancer and passive smoking. Int J Cancer 27:1.

Tulinius H, Day NE, Bjarnason O et al (1982) Familial breast cancer in Iceland. Int J Cancer 29:365.

Vena JE (1982) Air pollution as a risk factor in lung cancer. Amer J Epidemiol 116:42.

Waterhouse JAH, Muir CS, Correa, P & Powell J (eds) (1976) "Cancer Incidence in Five Continents" Vol III, Lyon, International Agency for Research on Cancer (IARC Scientific Publications No 15).

Waterhouse JAH, Muir CS, Powell J, Shanmugaratnam K (eds) (1982) "Cancer Incidence in Five Continents", Vol IV, Lyon, International Agency for Research on Cancer (IARC Scientific Publications No 42).

Wynder EL, Gori GB (1977) Contribution of the environment to cancer incidence: An epidemiologic exercise. J Natl Cancer Inst 58:825.

Wynder EL, Graham EA (1950) Tobacco smoking as a possible etiologic factor in bronchiogenic carcinoma. A study of six hundred and eighty-four proved cases. JAMA 143:329.

Yaker A & Dekkar N (1980) Profile de la morbidite cancereuse en Algerie 1966-1975. Algiers, Editions SNGD.

13th International Cancer Congress, Part A
Current Perspectives in Cancer, pages 107–131
© 1983 Alan R. Liss, Inc., 150 Fifth Avenue, New York, NY 10011

RECENT PROGRESS IN RADIATION ONCOLOGY

Maurice Tubiana, M.D.

Institut Gustave-Roussy

94800 Villejuif (France)

Twenty years ago in Moscow during the 8th International Cancer Congress I had the privilege of delivering a
lecture on radiation therapy (RT) (Tubiana 1964). It is
indeed a great honor that 2 decades later, I am again asked
to address this same topic.

Currently, like 2 decades ago, RT is one of the most
important methods of treatment of solid tumors. In England,
France and Canada about half of patients with solid tumors
receive RT and half surgery; in addition about half of those
patients who are cured of their solid tumors have been treated by RT. In the U.S. these proportions are significantly
lower.

During these 2 decades RT did not standstill. Like
medical oncology, it has evolved considerably. With improved
equipment it has become more effective and in addition it
has become increasingly integrated with surgery and chemotherapy (CT) in combined treatment protocols.

To better understand the present achievements of RT,
I would like first to review it from an historical perspective.

HISTORY OF RT

The Pioneers 1897-1919
The history of RT began almost immediately after the
discoveries of X Ray by Roentgen, radioactivity by Becquerel,
and Radium by the Curies.

Because the initial response of several types of cancers was so dramatic, this new form of therapy was greated
with considerable enthusiasm. A few years later, however,
there followed a wave of disillusionement. At this time the
massive dose treatments used caused a high rate of mortality,
while the results were at best palliative. These findings
led many physicians to conclude that RT had very little
curative potential. It is unfortunate that despite the
results which have since been obtained, vestiges of this
misconception persist even to-day.

What is most remarkable is that the pioneers were not
discouraged despite the unreliability of the X-ray tubes,
the high incidence of tumor recurrence, the severe injuries
to the normal tissues, and, in addition, the substantial
radiation toxicity to which the doctors and the technicians
were exposed during treatment.

However already at this time a few inspired researchers
(such as Bergonié and Tribondeau) were able to correlate
the responses of several types of normal tissues with their
rate of proliferation.

The Birth of Modern RT
Fractionation. Modern RT was born immediately after
the first world war. In 1919 Marie Curie, with the financial
help of the Rockfeller Foundation and of the Rothschild
family, created at the Radium Institute in Paris a wing
devoted to the development of experimental and clinical
radiotherapy.

There, in the 1920's, a team of young physicians, biologists and physicists headed by Regaud (1922, 1930) began
a series of experimental studies and clinical investigations.
Soon they discovered that fractionation improved the therapeutic ratio since the normal tissue was able to tolerate
much higher doses while at the same time the effect on the
tumor was much greater.

For their studies on fractionation, one of the early
models which they employed was the testis of the ram. They
observed that by the administration of successive daily doses
of fractionated RT, they were able to permanently eradicate
spermatogenesis without inducing intolerable injury to the
overlying skin. This finding contrasted strongly with the
results obtained with a single dose of RT if the dose admi-

nistered was high enough to eradicate spermatogenesis, it always caused severe skin injury (Regaud 1922).

While the relevance of this model to clinical RT may be questionned, these experimental data clearly showed that a differential effect on 2 tissues can be modulated by fractionation. Moreover they put the emphasis on the problem that matters : the tolerance of normal tissues. The clinical observations were so meticulously and so accurately made that within a few years, Regaud was able to define an optimal regimen of fraction which was soon universally used and still remains unchallenged. Indeed several attempts with other regimens have resulted in a higher incidence of late effects.

Recently, progress in understanding the radiobiological bases of fractionation have led to studies with multiple daily fractions, the preliminary results of which are promising (Dutreix et al. 1982). These new regimens in particular may facilitate combination of RT with drugs as well as the use of radiosensitizers (Tubiana et al. 1982).

Clinical dosimetry. A second important step was the measurement of dose distribution within the patient : several investigators, in particular the group of R. Paterson (1948) at Manchester, developed clinical dosimetry. The impact on beam RT and on Radium therapy was considerable. It became possible to study the dose-effect relationship for both tumor control and for injury to the normal surrounding tissues. Hence radiotherapists came to understand the importance of precise delivery of a cancericidal dose to the whole of the tumor while sparing as much of the surrounding normal tissues as possible.

At this time were introduced the philosophy of accepted risk and the concept of optimum dose, that is the dose which gives the highest incidence of tumor control with the lowest rate of severe complications. This concept was later substantiated by several clinical studies which showed that the numerical value of the optimum dose varies with the site of the tumor, its size, its histologic type and the technique of radiotherapy, in particular the size of the field.

The Mature Phase 1955-1980
Technical achievements : the megavoltage era. After the second world war several technical advances enabled RT to fulfill the promise of the preceding decades.

The high energy beams generated by telecobalt units, betatron, and linear accelerators liberated RT from the constraints of skin and superficial tissue reactions. Their high penetration made it possible to deliver sufficient doses to deep-seated tumors anywhere in the body.

Moreover, these beams have sharply defined edges which allow for treatment of lesions located near critical tissues, such as the eye. It is also possible to shape the beam with lead shields, filter wedges, and compensators, and thus to use large, complex fields tailored to the needs of the individual patient, such as the mantle field introduced by H.S. Kaplan (1966).

Computer dosimetry enabled mapping of the dose-distribution, not only in the plane through the center of the tumor, but also in any other parallel or perpendicular plane. Three dimensional display of the dose is becoming possible, a technique which will further ensure the precision and adequacy of dose distribution within the irradiated body.

Tumor localization is a prerequisite for precise RT. New tools such as C.T. scan, echography, emission tomoscintigraphy and more recently RMN have all dramatically improved the quality of tumordelineation, which in turn has resulted in much better treatment protocols. Since a small geographic miss or an underdosage to a small part of the tumor should lead to local failures, one hopes that these new imaging techniques will result in an increased incidence of tumor control and perhaps even a decreased incidence of injury to critical normal tissues. In our experience, at Villejuif, following a C.T. scan in about 15 % the beam size had to be enlarged in order to encompass all of the tumor while in about 15 % of the patients it was possible to reduce the field and thus to spare normal tissues.

The replacement of Radium by radioactive isotopes such as iridium wires and cesium seeds was another major advance which was particularly pioneered in France by B. Pierquin et al. (1978). In conjunction with afterloading techniques and computer dosimetry these artificial isotopes have greatly improved the efficacy of interstitial and intracavitary therapy. These modalities permit the intense, highly localized deposition of ionizing radiation in tissues seated deep within the body. These techniques are particularly useful in the treatment of carcinoma of the cervix, the bladder, and

the oral cavity. For example at Villejuif when Radium was
replaced by Iridium wires the survival rate of patients
with cancer of the anterior portion of the tongue has markedly increased from 18 % at 5 years for the 162 patients treated between 1960 and 1965 to 50 % at 5 years for the 161
patients treated between 1971 and 1973. The improvement is
particularly striking for stages I and II but it is also
noticeable in stage III, no improvement was observed in patients with stage IV disease (Richard et al., unpublished
data, Villejuif).

Proton beam RT and intraoperative radiotherapy represent promising avenues for research. Proton beam is probably
the ultimate in dose distribution and is currently investigated at Boston by H. Suit, Goiten et al. Intraoperative RT
has been pioneered in Japan (Abe, Takahashi 1981) and the
U.S. (Goldson 1981). With it 15 to 20 Gy can be delivered
via an electron beam to large tumors which are impossible to
resect completely. Subsequently post operative RT is performed.

Quality control. These technical refinements and the
highly-sophisticated RT that is being delivered in the large
specialized centers should not hide the fact that even in the
most industrialized countries the quality of the RT is not
the same in all centers.

Several muticenter cooperative trials performed in U.S.
and in Europe, have revealed that in some departments the
quality of the treatment technique was of questionable value.

In this context I quote the paragraph from a recent
report of the Gynecology Oncology Group which deals with
radiation technique : "Possibly the greatest major drawback
in this whole study was the fact that total abdominal radiation was not given for one-third of the patients as called
for in the protocol. A review of portal films indicates that
the upper magin fell below the diaphragms, and restricted
lateral margins left gutters of the abdomen on each side
untreated ; the lower margin fell short of the most inferior
portion of the pelvic cavity. In a few cases, there was apparent excessive blocking of liver and kidneys ... A lesson was
learned ... all therapy may not be as ideal as it is supposed
to be" (Lewis 1977).

In the U.S. an extensive survey has recently examined
the national profile of RT practice (Kramer 1981). Ten disease

sites were studied in which RT has an important therapeutic
role and for which a consensus of best management could be
obtained. A statistically valid sample of the RT facilities
in the U.S. was developed and a survey of these institutions
was carried out. How well each facility complied with the
established criteria for both the initial work-up and for
the treatment of each tumor type was analyzed. Complete
compliance with the study criteria, was scored as 100 and
lesser compliance by smaller numbers. It was observed that
compliance was much better in training institutions than in
non-training ones and in large institutions than in small
ones (fewer than 275 new patients per year). In addition
some important procedures were not carried out as frequently
as expected.

The outcome of the patients treated was also followed
and additional comparative surveys were performed for each
disease in the five institutions selected by virtue of the
largest annual experience in that particular disease. To
illustrate the findings of this study, I shall take as an
example carcinoma of the cervix. The absence of treatment
simulation, daily dose fractions exceeding 2 Gy, and a high
patient load per therapist were all associated with a significantly increased complication rate. In each stage the long
term results were significantly better in the five large
institutions. This underlines the importance of careful treatment technique. Failure to combine intracavitary irradiation
with beam therapy appears to be responsible, at least in part,
for the lower success obtained in the national practice. In
the five larger institutions, the amount of radiation given
to both central and lateral dose points was higher ; the
rate of pelvic control was better and, although the complication rate was higher, the proportion of survivors who
developed complications was identical in the two groups.

Similar data are available for nine other sites and
all of these data point out that major progress would result
from improving the quality of treatment up to the level of
those facilities with large annual experience.

The results of this survey should not lead us to think
that RT is poorer in the U.S. than in other parts of the
world. It is likely that a similar survey carried out in
other western countries would give similar or less satisfactory results. Indeed, typical results from the U.S. compare
favorably with the results from around the world. Moreover,

world wide surveys show a wide spread of RT results among different institutions.

Three major conclusions can be drawn from these studies :
1) The technique of treatment has a major impact on long term results. Quality control studies should be performed in each country and for each oncological speciality. Even in the most advanced countries there are opportunities for improvement. A major advance in RT results could be achieved simply by more widespread use of refined conventional techniques.
2) Teaching, training, and, for practicing radiotherapists, continuing education, are of paramount importance.
3) Large annual experience is a major factor in the quality of the results.

Although much remains to be done, it should be pointed out that the situation is slowly improving. Over the past three decades, a steady improvement in survival rates has been observed for all cancers treated by RT. For example, in 30 years the 5-year survival rate of cervix carcinoma (Kottmeier 1970) has increased from 36.9 % up to 52.2 % (results from 124 institutes in 24 countries, all stages), no doubt in large part due to improved radiotherapy techniques.
For Hodgkin's disease the progress is even more dramatic. It is also considerable for several other tumors, notably head and neck, and prostate cancer.

The impact of radiobiology. Since its onset, RT has had close links with radiobiology. Until the mid-century however radiobiology was purely descriptive, consisting largely of the morphological description of radiation damage. While these studies were interesting, they did not explain either how ionizing radiations could eradicate a malignant tumor without destroying the normal supporting tissues, or even the dose-effect relationships. Indeed, the radiobiological foundations of RT remained largely unexplored until about 25 years ago when, for the first time, the development of new techniques for the clonal cultivation of mammalian cells in vitro permitted quantitative analyses of the effect of radiation dosage (Puck and Marcus 1956). Following fractionated irradiation it can be considered as a first approximation that the cell survival curve is essentially a simple exponential function, therefore it takes the same amount of irradiation to deplete the same percentage of surviving

cells. Cell killing is a random event which is a reflection
of whether or not irreparable lethal damage has been caused
to the cell DNA. Similar survival curves have been obtained
for most antitumor drugs.

Let us examine the clinical implications of cell survival curves.

a - In 1966 we showed that regression of a tumor is a
complex phenomenon which is the result of 3 mechanisms : cell
killing, rate of dead cell removal, and repopulation (Tubiana
et al. 1968). A partial regression is generally defined as a
50 % reduction in tumor size. At a first approximation this
corresponds to the death of 50 % of ·the cells. If this is
obtained with a dose D_{50} total clinical disappearance of a
tumor of 100 g that is 10^{10} cells (complete regression) requires that at least 999 cells out of 1 000 are killed, as
a lump of 100 mg is no longer detectable ; this is obtained
with a dose 10 times larger : 10 D_{50}. If all the tumor cells
were clonogenic the cure of a tumor of 100 g would require
a dose equal to 36 D_{50}. If only 1 % of the tumor cells are
clonogenic, which appears more likely, then a dose 30A would
suffice. Whatever the precise proportion of clonogenic cells
the important point is that the dose needed to cure a tumor
is approximately 30 times larger than the dose which achieves
a significant partial regression and at least 3 times larger
than the dose which achieves a complete clinical remission.
As the survival of one clonogenic cell is sufficient to cause
a recurrence, it is easy to understand why although it may
have some relationship with patient cure, complete remission
does not reliably predict such an event.

b - It has long been known that bulky tumors require
higher radiation doses for control than do smaller ones. Cell
survival curves have helped to understand the relationships
between RT dose and tumor volume. If a full RT dose is required to control the primary tumor, for example a dose 30A corresponding to 9 logs of cell kill, then 2/3 of this dose or
20A, i.e. 6 logs of cell kill, would eliminate lumps 1 000
times smaller in volume, i.e. 10 times smaller in diameter.
For example if 66 Gy are required to control a lump with a
diameter of 4 cm, 44 Gy will sterilize the largest occult
metastatic focus (diameter 4 mm) (Fletcher 1973).

1) The concept of treatment of occult disease by relatively small doses, which was developed by Fletcher (1973,
1975, 1980), is of fundamental importance since 45 Gy is well
tolerated by normal tissues whereas 65 Gy or higher doses
may induce sequellae.

2) It provides a rationale for the shrinking field technique, introduced long ago by Baclesse, and the widely-used booster technique.

3) A few decades ago elective post-operative irradiation was used infrequently because the prevailing concept held that one should wait for recurrence in order to have something tangible to irradiate. When it was recognized that higher doses are required to eradicate gross masses than subclinical disease, the use of prophylactic irradiation of clinically univolved areas at a risk of containing occult deposits was greatly enhanced. The analysis of the clinical data soon substantiated this concept and this method has become widely used with excellent clinical results (Fletcher 1980).

4) More recently prophylactic bilateral pulmonary irradiation was used to control micrometastases (Breur et al. 1978). In this treatment no more than 20 Gy could be delivered because of the risk of late effects. Nevertheless in the EORTC osteosarcoma trial this dose proved to be sufficient to check neoplastic microfoci up to about 10^6 cells (1 cubic millimeter). This result is better than expected (Tubiana 1982) and suggests that such other factors as absence of anoxic cells and a rapid rate of cell proliferation may contribute to the high radiosensitivity of these small cell aggregates, ideas consistent with the experimental data.

5) The understanding of the dose cell survival relationship also gave a rationale for combining irradiation and surgery. Recurrence following surgery is due to microscopic disease which was not removed despite radical and mutilating procedures. The incidence of failure following RT increases with the volume of the tumor despite high doses which caused late severe effects. It follows that the 2 treatment modalities are complementary : surgical excision of the gross masses and relatively modest doses of RT to eradicate the surrounding subclinical disease (Fletcher 1980). Such a procedure is now used for a number of cancer sites and this combination of 2 less than radical procedures not only increases survival rates but in addition improves markedly the quality of life. Conservative treatment of small breast cancer is a good example of this approach.

Baclesse first demonstrated in 1936 that breast cancer can be cured by RT alone. The high doses necessary, however, induced severe breast fibrosis, so the cosmetic results were unsatisfactory. The early works of R. Calle (1978), V. Peters

(1977), Mustakallio (1972), on combination of lumpectomy and
RT as well as the concept of occult disease introduced by
G. Fletcher (1975) gave a rationale to a conservative approach.
A first clinical trial (Atkins et al. 1972) comparing radical
surgery and tumorectomy + RT was unsuccessful because the
irradiation dose was too low (35 Gy) and unable to control
palpable axillary lymph nodes. Two subsequent trials, those
of Veronesi et al. (1981) on quadrantectomy, and of D.
Sarrazin et al. (1980) on tumorectomy, did demonstrate that
for breast tumors, the survival rates obtained with a conservative approach were as good as those of radical mastectomy.
In addition, with tumorectomy the cosmetic results were excellent in over 80 % of the patients. Thus the unambiguous demonstration of the validity of this method took about 4 decades.

In parallel it was shown that irradiation of the internal mammary chain is just as efficient as is radical dissection and it represents a useful procedure for tumors of the
inner quadrants (Sarrazin et al. 1982).

In large head and neck tumors, combination of RT and
surgery also contributed to both an increase in survival
rate and a reduction in patient mutilation as well as a
conservation of the function.

Combination of RT and chemotherapy (CT). RT is a regional treatment which can control tumor masses up to several
centimeters in diameter, CT is a systemic treatment but for
most solid tumors it cannot control neoplastic aggregates of
more than a few millimeters in diameter. Hence the 2 modalities are complementary. Their combination has two purposes :
1) Spatial cooperation. The two target volumes are
different :
- CT is used to control disseminated disease while RT is
directed against localized tumors ;
- or RT is used for sanctuaries in which the drug concentration is low, i.e. brain in acute leukemia.

In these situations, the chance for cure is equal to
that of the less effective of the 2 treatments.
2) The two modalities both aim at eradication of the
primary tumor. Although this method has strong experimental
basis, most of the clinical results have been disappointing.
As we have seen, a radiation dose of approximately 30 D_{50}
is required to control a tumor when treated by RT solely,
it follows that when CT is used first and has been able to

decrease :
- the tumor volume by half, the necessary RT dose is 29 D_{50}
- the tumor diameter by half, the necessary RT dose is 26 D_{50}.

It is only when CT has produced a complete disappearance of the tumor that RT given to treat the areas of the original gross mass to eradicate the remaining subclinical disease can be reduced to 20 D_{50}.

Even when this is the case, combination of RT + CT is useful only if the sum of the effects of the 2 modalities is less for the normal tissues than for the tumor. Concomitant administration of drugs and ionizing radiation is generally as effective on normal tissues as on the tumor. This appears to be the cause of the failures of concomitant administration of CT + RT for example in head and neck tumors (Cachin et al. 1977). This once more underlines the importance of normal tissue tolerance, and shows that a small decrease in radiation dose which is tolerated may outweigh a notable killing effect.

Sequential administration is currently preferred because a short gap gives the normal tissues time to repair between the two modalities. However early administration of both modalities is advisable because the proliferation of the cells which are not reached by or are resistant to one of the treatment forms is prevented. In order to reconcile the needs for early administration of both agents and to accomplish their sequential administration, RT and CT can be laternated. With such a schedule the rythm of CT is not altered. Good results have been obtained in experimental tumors (Looney et al. 1981). We have use this format in oat cell carcinoma of the lung and in non-Hodgkin lymphoma and the clinical results look promising (Tubiana, Arriagada et al. 1982).

With the advent of new drugs which are more effective and with less cross-toxicity, such new strategies for solid tumors should be investigated and tested. It is only by trial and error, step by step, that progress in this field will be achieved.

Hyperthermia. In the search for agents without cross toxicity and without cross resistance to ionizing radiation, hyperthermia seems to be a good candidate. Moreover it is a modality which is more effective on large tumors than on small ones because the poor average perfusion which is a major

drawback to both RT and CT actually becomes advantageous.
Less heat is carried away and the temperature rises more in
the tumor than in sourrounding normal tissues. A few thousand
patients have been treated and some of the tumor responses
are promising. However the clinical use of hyperthermia is
hampered by technical problems : there is no good way of
delivering the heat deep in the tissues ; and dosimetry is
poor. In this context interstitial hyperthermia probably has
a great future.

The Future : and Now Where ?
        The first question we must ask is will improved local
tumor control which results from an increase in the efficacy
of therapy directed at the primary tumor be translated to
improved long-term survival ?

        This question is a fundamental one. Most of the primary
tumors which are not controlled by RT are bulky tumors. If
those patients with uncontrolled tumors already have occult
metastases at the time of treatment, a gain in local control
frequency would only result in an increased incidence of death
due to distant metastases. However studies about the natural
history of human tumors suggest that a noticeable proportion
of relatively large tumors have not yet metastasized
(Tubiana 1982).

        Moreover it should be pointed out that much experimen-
tal data support the notion that those mice with recurrent
carcinoma have a higher incidence of distant metastases
(Sheldon et al. 1974; Suit 1982; Romsdahl et al. 1961).
Anderson and Dische (1981) have analysed the data from two
series of patients with bladder cancer and cervical carcinoma
randomized to receive either RT in hyperbaric oxygen or in
air. The results show that metastasis is very frequent in
those patients with uncontrolled or recurrent local tumors.
Indeed life table analysis suggests that virtually all patients with local failure would have shown distant metastasis
had they survived long enough. Stratification analyses were
made with regard to the various stages of disease, the histo-
logical grade of tumors, and the size of primary tumors. In
all subgroups primary tumor control is associated with a lower
incidence of metastasis in the subsequent years when compared
with those patients whose tumor is never controlled or controlled only for a period of time. A possible explanation for this
correlation is that a tumor which is highly radiosensitive
may also have a diminished tendency to show distant metastasis.

Clinical experience and cell kinetic studies suggest the opposite association. Anaplastic tumors as well as tumors with a high labeling index commonly respond well to RT but often show remote metastasis at an early date (Tubiana et al. 1981). Thus the more likely interpretation for the observed difference is that of metastatic spread originates from persistent or recurrent tumor, and therefore local control of primary tumor is likely to prevent at least some of the metastatic disease. This is confirmed by the analysis of the conservative breast cancer trial of Atkins et al. (1972). In this trial the doses to the breast and the axilla were too low and the incidence of local recurrence and of metastasis was higher than in the patients treated by radical mastectomy.

H. Suit (1982) attempted to estimate the extent of this prevention. He observed that for several sites salvage treatment for local failures either by surgery or radiation resulted in worthwhile long term disease free survival. This suggests that there is a potential for an increase in survival with more effective local treatment. Review of clinical studies was based on detailed analysis of causes of failure.

The increase in survival of patients by employing a treatment method which yields a 100 % local control rate was estimated by assuming that the rates of death due to distant metastasis among patients who achieved a control of their primary tumor by conventional treatment would apply to the patients achieving local control by the new method. Under this assumption Suit calculated that for cervix cancers the 5-year survival rates would increase from 65 % to 85 %. With a more conservative assumption the increase would be from 65 % to 75 %.

For cancer of the oral cavity and oropharynx the increase would be from 37 % to 51 %. By and large, these predicted increases in survivors due to improved local treatment methods compare favourably with those which have been achieved or could be achieved by improving treatment of occult metastases. Research in RT is fully deserved and should be pursued and enlarged.

What are currently the main avenues for research in RT?

Radioresistance of human tumors. In order to improve local control rates we must identify the causes of failures.

Since the onset of RT it was recognized that human tumors varied widely in their radiosensitivity.

In this context tumors were regarded as radiosensitive if they responded rapidly to modest doses of ionizing radiations while radioresistant tumors showed little or no apparent response to even highest doses. As we have seen, it was later discovered that the early shrinkage of a tumor under treatment indicated a rapid cell turnover rate, a response which does not necessarily correlate with radiocurability. Nevertheless the fact remains that among tumors of the same size, some can be eradicated by doses of the order of 40 to 60 Gy while others do not respond to doses as high as 80 Gy. Moreover there is an obvious correlation between the histologic type of a tumor and its radiocurability. Tumors of the GI tract for example are more resistant than are embryonal tumors such as seminoma or nephroblastoma.

Within one histologic type however there is a wide range of probability of tumor control.

While there are many reasons why a tumor may be radioresistant, the relevant causes in clinical radiotherapy are still unclear.

Hypoxia. Gray et al. (1953) showed that in experimental tumors hypoxia was a major factor in radioresistance. This has opened a whole line of experimental and clinical research. The main methods which were tested were :
- Hyperbaric oxygen tanks,
- High LET particle therapy, in particular neutrons,
- Electron affinic hypoxic cell radiosensitizers.
The improvement in local control obtained with these three methods are yet not convincing.

The head and neck trials carried out with hyperbaric oxygen suggest a small but significant oxygen effect in particular for certain tumors of medium size i.e. T3 glottic carcinoma or oral carcinoma of 2 to 5 cm diameter. In carcinoma of the cervix however any advantage of hyperbaric oxygen over conventional fractionation in air is negligible. As this procedure is time consuming and somewhat cumbersome its use is becoming less and less frequent (Henk 1981).

Particle therapy. Two dozen centers in ten countries are conducting neutron trials. The results of these trials

are conflicting. One center has shown a significant advantage
of neutron particles over photons for head and neck tumors
but doubts have been raised as to whether the results obtained
in the control arm are as good as expected. Other data showed
no evidence of improvement with neutron therapy (Fowler 1981).

It should be pointed out however that most of the cyclotrons which are currently used for RT are physicist cyclotrons in which the facilities for human therapy are far from
optimal. It will probably be another decade before results
from therapy using the new medical cyclotrons becomes available.

Radiosensitizers. Approximately fifteen phase 2 and
ten phase 3 controlled clinical trials have been just termi-
nated in Europe, and in the U.S., or are currently on-going.
None of the available results show any significant benefit
from the use of radiosensitizers. However their neurotoxicity
has been greater than expected, a result which has limited
the amount of sensitizer which could be given to the patients.
Attempts to find less neurotoxic sensitizers are underway and
some of them have already given promising results in experimental animals (Adams et al. 1982).

Despite the technical problems which may to some extent
be responsible for the lack of success, the absence of a
clear-cut benefit from the methods which have been tried
raises a basic question : is hypoxia a cause of radioresistance ? Since there is overhelming circumstantial evidence
that hypoxic cells exist in most human tumors (Bush et al.
1978) it must be assumed that when human tumors are controlled
by RT, the process of reoxygenation during therapy has circum-
vented the radioresistance of hypoxic cells. In this context
the results of the Capetown trial are particularly valuable
because it compared conventional and short, i.e. 27 and 10
fraction schemes in both oxygen and air. Oxygen improved the
results significantly with 10 fractions but not with 27. Twenty seven fractions however gave a lower morbidity than 10
fractions (Bennett 1978). Thus courses of RT as long as 6 or
7 weeks allows time for reoxygenation of most tumors.

Nevertheless it remains probable that some treatment
failures with conventional techniques can be attributed to
failure of reoxygenation but in the current trials with neutrons or sensitizers :
1) those tumors which do not reoxygenate are too heavily

diluted with tumors that do reoxygenate and so do not need
neutrons or radiosensitizers,
2) only a small proportion of them are controlled with the
new methods in their present status.

This underlines the need for 1) less toxic radiosensitizers and better technique with heavy particles, 2) an
effort to identify those tumors which do require some help
in the elimination of hypoxic cells.

Moreover heavy particles deserve further study because
1) neutrons in addition to oxygen effect may have other radiobiologic therapeutic advantages in particular for tumors with
a low proliferative potential, 2) protons, heavy ions and
negative pi mesons provide excellent dose distribution at
depth in tissue.

Tumor cell kinetics. Tumor cell proliferation influences
clinical radioresistance in three ways :
1) Rapid repopulation during a conventional fractionated RT.
This has been observed in several experimental tumors
(Barendsen et al. 1970; Tubiana et al. 1968). Clinical support
for these mechanisms was provided by studies in Burkitt's
lymphoma (Norin 1977). In this disease better results were
obtained with short overall time treatment schedules with
three fractions per day than with regular daily fractionation.

Although it is unlikely that in most human tumors rapid
repopulation may be a cause of radioresistance, an effort
should be made to identify those tumors with rapid repopulation rate during fractionated radiotherapy. We already know
that excessively protracted or split course regimens might
be less effective than conventional ones and this demonstrates that repopulation may play a role (Tubiana 1982).
2) Slow growing tumors are less radiosensitive. This might
be due to two factors : a) slow clearance of killed cells
which may interfere with reoxygenation ; b) repair of potential lethal damage which is more effective in non-dividing
cells. For example experimental data have shown that it is
more effective in large tumors in which there is a large
proportion of quiescent cells than in small tumors in which
most of the cells are proliferating (Little et al. 1973).
3) Proportion of clonogenic cells. In experimental tumors
assays of cellular reproductive integrity have shown that
the proportion of cells capable of regenerating the tumor
may range from 1 in 2 to 1 in 10^4 cells. While estimates of

the proportion of clonogenic cells in human tumors are impre-
cise, it has been suggested to be 1 in 10^2 to 10^4 cells.
Obviously a high proportion of clonogenic cells should be
correlated with a high radioresistance.

In conclusion cell kinetics may play a role in the
radioresistance of some tumors, but it is still difficult
to accurately assess its importance.

Intrinsic radioresistance. It has long been assumed
that all mammalian cells whether normal or neoplastic have
similar radiosensitivities.

With the introduction of more accurate cell-survival
curves and operational methods to assay cell survival, this
concept has recently been challenged. Barendsen has shown
that the cell survival curves for various types of normal
cells have different initial slopes (1982). These differences
may explain varying amount of acute and late effects which
have long been observed using different fractionation regimens.

The data obtained by Fertil and Malaise (1981) with
several human neoplastic cell lines strongly suggest that
differences in the surviving fraction after doses of 2 Gy
may help to explain the different radiation dosage required
for control of various human cancers. The clinical implications of variations in intrinsic radioresistance have long
been overlooked whereas this is an important avenue for
research because it may lead to the early identification of
radioresistant tumors and a better understanding of the relationship between radioresistance and histologic cell type.

In conclusion several factors are probably involved in
clinical radioresistance. We now have available powerful
tools which may soon : 1) help to establish the respective
role of each of these factors, 2) identify those tumors in
which they are of major importance.

Better knowledge of the pattern of spread of the different type of cancer arising in a variety of sites. Knowledge
on pathways of spread has been obtained by sustained and
cooperative efforts of radiotherapists with surgeons, pathologists and diagnosticians. The goal of such studies is to
develop new therapeutic strategies linked to the natural
history of the corresponding neoplasms.

While these studies could be illustrated by several cancer types I shall focus on one example, that of ovarian carcinoma.

At the Princess Margaret Hospital in Toronto following surgery for localized disease patients were randomized, to receive either pelvic irradiation or observation only (Dembo, Bush 1982). The frequency of relapse did not differ significantly between the two groups. This was not due to the inefficacy of RT but to the insufficiency of pelvic irradiation alone and indeed the sites of relapse extended throughout the whole of the peritoneal cavity. This suggested that irradiation not confined to the pelvis but extended to the entire peritoneal cavity was needed. The first attempts with this technique were not satisfactory because the liver and kidneys were shielded to avoid organ toxicity. When it was recognized that the drainage of fluid and cells from the peritoneal cavity took place via the diaphragmatic lymphatics, the Stanford group (Glatstein et al. 1977) and the Toronto group elected to encompass the entire diaphragm in the treatment portal without liver shielding. To accomplish this, a radiation dose within liver tolerance was required. This new strategy has been successful, and, in patients with no evident residual tumor, a relatively small dose (22.5 Gy) yielded significantly better results than pelvic irradiation alone or combined with chlorambucil. However patients with macroscopic residum were not controlled by those doses. A multivariate analysis was able to identify several groups of patients : those who do not need post-operative RT, those who can be controlled by abdominopelvic RT and those for whom this modality is insufficient and for whom attempts are being made to combine CT and subsequent RT. This study illustrates one of the main trends of modern RT : individualization of cancer treatment.

Individualization of cancer treatment. Role of prognostic factors. In the last decade it has become increasingly clear that while still useful, the anatomical stage is not a totally sufficient method for describing patient groups either for purposes of prognostication or for choice of therapy.

To illustrate this point I shall take two examples. In Hodgkin's disease the results of RT in stage II patients are strongly correlated with two prognostic factors : 1) the erythrocyte sedimentation rate (ESR) ; 2) the number of involved lymphatic node areas.

Thus, one can identify among patients with stage II disease subsets for whom RT gives either excellent or wholly insufficient results (Tubiana et al. 1979; Tubiana et al. 1981). Clinically such prognostic factors are important because the combination of RT and chemotherapy carries with it risks of severe late effects on the gonads as well as a increased incidence of secondary cancer.

In breast cancer for tumors of the same size and without palpable axillary lymph nodes the outcome is influenced by several prognostic factors such as histologic grade and labeling index, histologic involvement of axillary lymph nodes, localization of the tumor to the inner or outer quadrants of the breast. In some of the subgroups of patients postoperative RT does not seem warranted while it is of clinical benefit in others. Similarly the risk of occult remote metastases is high in some subsets of patients and low in others (Sarrazin et al. 1982).

It has always been a dream to tailor a treatment to the individual characteristics of the tumor and the patient. We are now reaching the point where this is becoming feasible in clinical practice.

Generalized disease - Total body irradiation. Approximately 2/3 of patients who die from their cancer die from metastatic disease.

We have already seen that RT could prevent some of this spread by more effective treatment of the primary cancer or by irradiation of occult metastases (bilateral lung irradiation).

However an important question is what could RT offer to patients with clinical metastatic disease ? It can offer:
1 - Palliation. RT exerts a powerful action against pain ;
2 - For cancer with a high radiosensitivity and a high chemosensitivity (such as lymphoma, embryonal tumors, oat cell carcinoma), the combination of RT for gross disease plus CT for occult metastasis could give good results but the limiting factor in these treatments is the risk of blood aplasia.

Bone marrow grafting might offer an answer to this problem. Let us assume that this is feasible. Extended field

RT can be used to deliver up to 20-25 Gy on a large target volumes. If chemotherapy is then added, one could hope to control cell aggregates up to 10^6-10^7 cells which would encompass most occult disease. Moreover booster could be theoretically used on detectable disease, and the cure of a wide spectrum disseminated cancer might become a reality.

What type of bone marrow transplantation should be used? Autologous marrow engraftment has a higher success of marrow engraftment, avoids graft versus host disease (GVH), and reduces the risk of secondary infection. However its main restriction is, of course, the potential concomitant transplantation of neoplastic cells.

It is therefore restricted to cancer in which the risk of bone marrow involvement is small or in which it is possible to segregate tumor cells from bone marrow hemopoietic stem cells. This might be achieved by separation (Rubin et al. 1981) or selective killing of neoplastic cells. Moreover when a sufficient quantity of marrow has been stored iterative graftings following iterative courses of treatment become conceivable.

The use of allograft after total body irradiation is justified when elimination of neoplastic from bone marrow is difficult or impossible, as for example in leukemia. Spectacular success has recently been obtained and the incidence of deaths caused by GVH has been markedly reduced. It might be further reduced in the near future by techniques such as elimination of the T-lymphocytes from the bone marrow graft. When this is achieved TBI + allograft might become more widely used in several diseases.

Total nodal irradiation offers an attracting alternate method for overcoming immunologic desfense prior to an allograft (Fuks et al. 1981). Moreover it might offer an efficient treatment for a wide spectrum of autoimmune diseases.

To-day some of these prospects may seem like science fiction, but I am convinced that we shall hear a lot about them at the next congress.

In conclusion RT lies at the cross roads of physics, radiobiology and oncology. During the past half century it has benefitted from the advances which have been made in physics and dosimetry as well as from many empirical clinical observations. It is now taking advantage of progress in the areas of radiobiology and oncology. However an integrated effort between radiotherapy, medical oncology, surgery and basic research is still required to take full advantage of the individual characteristics as well as the difference in natural history of the various types of human tumors. Meanwhile a close cooperation on an equality basis of the surgeon, the medical oncologist and the radiotherapist within multidisciplinary teams is the only way to offer to each patient the highest chance for cure with the smallest mutilation and at the smallest toxic cost.

References

Abe M, Takahashi M (1981). Intraoperative radiotherapy : the Japanese experience. Int J Radiat Oncol 7:863.

Adams GE, Sheldon PW, Stratford IJ (1982). How do we find better radiosensitizers. In Karcher KH et al. (eds): "Progress in Radio-Oncology II", New York: Raven Press.

Anderson P, Dische S (1981). Local tumor control and the subsequent incidence of distant metastatic disease. Int J Radiat Oncol 7:1645.

Atkins H, Hayward JL, Klugman DJ, Wayte AB (1972). Treatment of early breast cancer : a report after ten years of a clinical trial. Brit Med J 2:423.

Baclesse F, Ennuyer A, Cheguillaume J (1960). Est-on autorisé à pratiquer une tumorectomie simple suivie de radiothérapie en cas de tumeurs mammaires ? J Radiol Electrol Med Nucl 41:137.

Baclesse F (1965). Five-year results in 431 breast cancers treated solely by Roentgen Rays. Ann Surg 161:103.

Barendsen GW, Broerse JJ (1970). Experimental radiotherapy of a rat rhabdomyosarcoma. II - Effects of fractionated treatments. Europ J Cancer 6:89.

Barendsen GW (1982). Dose fractionation, dose rate and iso-effect relationship for normal tissue responses. Int J Radiat Oncol (in press).

Bennett MB (1978). The treatment of stage III squamous carcinoma of the cervix in air and hyperbaric oxygen. Br J Radiol 51:68.

Bergonié J, Tribondeau L (1906). Interprétation de quelques résultats de la radiothérapie et essai de fixation d'une technique rationnelle. C R Séances Acad Sci 143:983.

Breur K, Cohen P, Schweisguth O, Hart AMM (1978). Irradiation of the lungs as an adjuvant therapy of osteosarcoma of the limbs. An EORTC randomized study. Europ J Cancer

14:461.

Bush RS, Jenkin RDT, Allt WEC, Beale FA, Bean H, Dembo AJ, Pringle JF (1978). Definitive evidence of hypoxic cells influencing cure in cancer therapy. Br J Cancer 37:302.

Cachin Y, Jortay A, Sancho H, Eschwege F, Madelain M, Desaulty A, Gerard P (1977). Preliminary results of a randomized EORTC study comparing radiotherapy and concomitant Bleomycin to radiotherapy alone in epidermoid carcinomas of the oropharynx. Eur J Cancer 13:1389.

Calle R, Pilleron JP, Schlienger P, Vilcoq JR (1978). Conservative management of operable breast cancer. Ten years experience at the Foundation Curie. Cancer 42:2045.

Dembo AJ, Bush RS (1982). Radiation therapy of ovarian carcinoma. In Griffiths CT (ed): "Cancer Research and Treatment - Gynecological Malignancy I". Boston: M Nijhoff.

Dutreix J, Cosset JM, Eschwege F, Wambersie A (1982). Biological and therapeutic studies of multifractionation. In Karcher KH et al. (eds): "Progress in Radio-Oncology II", New York: Raven Press.

Fertil B, Malaise EP (1981). Inherent cellular radiosensitivity as a basic concept for human tumor radiotherapy. Int J Radiat Oncol 7:621.

Fletcher GH (1973). Clinical dose response curves of human malignant epithelial tumors. Brit J Radiol 46:1.

Fletcher GH, Shukovsky LJ (1975). The interplay of radiocurability and tolerance in the irradiation of human cancers. J Radiol Electrol 56:383.

Fletcher GH (1980). "Textbook of Radiotherapy". Philadelphia: Lea & Febiger.

Fowler JF (1981). "Nuclear Particles in Cancer Treatment". Bristol: Adam Hilger.

Fuks Z, Slavin S (1981). The use of total lymphoid irradiation as an immunosuppressive therapy for organ allotransplantation and autoimmune disease. Int J Radiat Oncol 7:79.

Glatstein E, Fuks Z, Bagshaw MA (1977). Diaphragmatic treatment in ovarian carcinoma: A new radiotherapeutic technique. Int J Radiat Oncol Biol Phys 2:357.

Goldson AL (1981). The outlook for intraoperative radiotherapy. Int J Radiat Oncol 7:979.

Gray LH, Conger AD, Ebert M, Hornsey S, Scott OCA (1953). The concentration of oxygen dissolved in tissues at the time of irradiation as a factor in radiotherapy. Brit J Radiol 26:638.

Hanks GE, Herring DF, Kramer S (1982). Pattern of care-outcome studies : Results of the national practice in cervix cancer. (submitted for publication).

Henk JM (1981). Does hyperbaric oxygen have a future in radiation therapy. Int J Radiat Oncol 7:1125.

Kaplan HS, Rosenberg SA (1966). Extended field radical radiotherapy in advanced Hodgkin's disease: short term results of 2 randomized clinical trials. Cancer Res 26:1268.

Kottmeier HL (1970). 15th Annual report on the results of treatment in carcinoma of the uterus, vagina and ovary: treatments in 1954-63.

Kramer S (1981). An overview of process and outcome data in the patterns of care study. Int J Radiat Oncol Biol Phys 7:795.

Lewis GC, Blessing J (1977). Ovarian cancer: Use of multiple modality programs involving surgery, radiation therapy and chemotherapy. Cancer 40:588.

Little JB, Hahn GM, Frindel E, Tubiana M (1973). Repair of potentially lethal radiation damage in vitro and in vivo. Radiology 106:689.

Looney WB, Ritenour ER, Hopkins HA (1981). Solid tumor models for the assessment of different treatment modalities: XVI sequential combined modality (cyclophosphamid-radiation) therapy. Cancer 47:860.

Mustakallio S (1972). Conservative treatment of breast carcinoma. Review of 25 years follow-up. Clin Radiol 23:110.

Norin T, Onyango J (1977). Radiotherapy in Burkitt's lymphoma: Conventional or superfractionated regime. Int J Radiat Oncol Biol Phys 2:399.

Paterson R (1948). "The treatment of Malignant Disease by Radium and X-Rays". London: Edward Arnold.

Peters MV (1977). Wedge resection with or without radiation in early breast cancer. Int J Radiat Oncol Biol Phys 2:1151.

Pierquin B, Mueller W, Baillet F, Maylin C, Raynal M, Otmezguine Y (1978). Radical radiation therapy for cancer of the breast. The experience of Creteil. In Vaeth JM et al. (eds): "Renaissance of interstitial brachytherapy", Basel: Karger, p 150.

Pierquin B, Dutreix A (1967). Toward a new system in Curietherapy. Brit J Radiol 40:184.

Pierquin B, Dutreix A, Paine CH, Chassagne D, Marinello G, Ash D (1978). The Paris System in interstitial radiation therapy. Acta Radiol Oncol 17:33.

Pierquin B, Chassagne D, Chahbazian CM, Wilson F (1978). "Brachytherapy". Saint-Louis (USA): Warreen Green.

Pierquin B (1982). Klaas Breur Memorial Lecture. E S T R O Londres, June 29, 1982.

Puck TT, Marcus PI (1956). Action of X-Rays on mammalian cells. J Exp Med 103:651.

Regaud C (1922). Influence de la durée d'irradiation sur les effets déterminés dans le testicule par le radium. CR Soc Biol (Paris) 86:787.

Regaud ·C (1930). Sur les principes radiophysiologiques de la radiothérapie des cancers. Acta Radiol (Stockholm) 11:456.

Romsdahl MD, Chu EW, Hume R, Smith RR (1961). The time of metastasis and release of circulating tumor cells as determined in an experimental system. Cancer 14:883.

Rubin P, Wheeler KT, Keng PC, Gregory PK, Croizat H (1981). The separation of a mixture of bone marrow stem cells from tumor cells. An essential step for autologous bone marrow transplantation. Int J Radiat Oncol 7:1405.

Sarrazin D, Tubiana M, Le M, Fontaine F, Arriagada R (1980). Conservative treatment of minimal breast cancer. In Mouridsen HT, Palshof T (eds): "Breast Cancer. Experimental and Clinical Aspects", Oxford: Pergamon Press, p 251.

Sarrazin D, Le M, Mouriesse H, Contesso G, Fontaine F, Arriagada R, Tubiana M (1982). Past and present radiotherapy studies for breast cancer carried out at Villejuif. Cancer Bulletin (in press).

Sheldon PW, Begg AC, Fowler JF, Lansley IF (1974). The incidence of lung metastases in C3H mice after treatment of implanted solid tumours with X-rays or surgery. Br J Cancer 30:342.

Suit HD, Sedlacek R, Gillette EL (1970). Examination for a correlation between probabilities of development of distant metastasis and of local recurrence. Radiology 95:189.

Suit H (1982). Potential for improving survival rates for the cancer patient by increasing the efficacy of treatment of the primary lesion.(submitted for publication).

Suit H, Goiten M, Munzenrider et al. (1982). Evaluation of the clinical applicability of proton beam in definition fractionated radiation therapy. (submitted for publication).

Tubiana M (1964). New methods of treatment in radiation therapy. Clinical Radiology 15:142.

Tubiana M, Frindel E, Malaise E (1968). The application of radiobiologic knowledge and cellular kinetics to radiation therapy. Am J Roentgenol 102:822.

Tubiana M, Henry-Amar M, Hayat M, Breur K, Van Der Werf Messing B, Burgers M (1979). Long-term results of the EORTC randomized study of irradiation and Vinblastine in clinical stages I and II of Hodgkin's disease. Europ J Cancer 15:645.

Tubiana M, Hayat M, Henry-Amar M, Breur K, Van Der Werf Messing B, Burgers M (1981). Five-year results of the EORTC randomized study of splenectomy and spleen irradia-

tion in clinical stages I and II of Hodgkin's disease.
Europ J Cancer 17:355.

Tubiana M, Arriagada R, Cosset JM (1982). New types of fractionation for optimization of combination of radiotherapy
and chemotherapy. In Kärcher KH, Kogelnik HD, Reinartz G
(eds): "Progress in Radio-Oncology II", New York: Raven
Press Pub, p 387.

Tubiana M, Péjovic MJ, Renaud A, Contesso G, Chavaudra N,
Gioanni J, Malaise EP (1981). Kinetic parameters and the
course of the disease in breast cancer. Cancer 47:937.

Tubiana M (1982). Cell kinetics and radiation oncology. Int
J Radiat Oncol 8:1471.

Veronesi U, Saccozzi R, Del Vecchio M, Banfi A, Clemente C,
De Lena M, Gallus G, Greco M, Luini A, Marubini E,
Muscolino G, Rilke F, Salvadori B, Zecchini A, Zucali R
(1981). Comparing radical mastectomy with quadrantectomy,
axillary dissection, and radiotherapy in patients with
small cancers of the breast. New England J of Med 305:6.

13th International Cancer Congress, Part A
Current Perspectives in Cancer, pages 133–139
© 1983 Alan R. Liss, Inc., 150 Fifth Avenue, New York, NY 10011

THE ROLE OF INTENSIVE CHEMORADIOTHERAPY AND MARROW
TRANSPLANTATION IN THE TREATMENT OF DISSEMINATED
MALIGNANT DISEASE

E. Donnall Thomas, M.D.

Professor of Medicine,
University of Washington School of Medicine,
Associate Director for Clinical Research,
Fred Hutchinson Cancer Research Center
Seattle, Washington 98104

The Seattle Marrow Transplant Team has now carried
out over 1200 transplants for hematologic diseases, and
marrow transplants are also being carried out in many
other transplant centers. The clinical achievements in
the field of marrow transplantation are the culmination
of more than 20 years of work by this and many other
groups studying the principles of transplantation
biology, tissue typing, supportive care of the patient
without marrow function, and pre- and post-marrow
grafting regimens (Thomas 1975). The basic concept of
marrow transplantation is rather simple. Malignant
cells are destroyed by high dose chemoradiotherapy
without regard for marrow toxicity because marrow
function is to be restored by transplantation of normal
marrow cells. A marrow graft includes not only the
marrow but also the lymphoid and monocyte-macrophage
systems (Thomas 1976) which may have an adverse effect
on any residual malignant cells. The normal marrow may
be the patient's own marrow which has been cryopreserved
(autologous transplant), an identical twin (syngeneic
transplant) or a donor compatible for the major histo-
compatibility complex, HLA (allogeneic transplant).

The first 110 patients transplanted in Seattle all
had acute leukemia in an endstage relapse state (Thomas
1977). They were prepared for transplantation with
cyclophosphamide followed by 1000 rad total body
irradiation and a marrow transplant from an HLA
identical sibling. This lethal dose of total body
irradiation was used to create "room" in the marrow

cavities and also to suppress the host immune system. In addition, irradiation has long been known to be an excellent method of killing malignant cells and it also penetrates the privileged sites such as the central nervous system and the testes. There were many early deaths from advanced illness and subsequent deaths from graft-versus-host disease (GVHD), opportunistic infection and recurrence of leukemia in this first group of patients. However, 7 patients with acute lymphocytic leukemia (ALL) and 6 patients with acute nonlymphocytic leukemia (ANL) are alive in unmaintained remission from 7 to 12 years later. Actuarial analysis of this survival curve demonstrates a flat longterm disease free plateau and provides evidence that these patients are indeed cured of their disease. Similarly, 8 of 34 patients with end-stage acute leukemia given syngeneic grafts are in remission 3 to 11 years after grafting (Fefer 1981).

Encouraged by these results, it therefore seemed justifiable to undertake transplantation at an earlier stage of the disease when the patient would be in a better condition. Twenty-two patients with ANL in first remission were treated with the same regimen and 12 are in continuing remission 4 to 6 years later (Thomas 1982a).

Transplant for patients with ANL in first relapse has resulted in 7 of 40 patients in remission beyond 2 years (18%) (Buckner 1982b). Transplantation in second or subsequent remission for patients with either ANL or ALL gives a long-term disease free survival of approximately 20-30% (Buckner 1982a; Clift 1982).

A study designed to compare the efficacy and toxicity of the 1000 rad regimen to a fractionated regimen consisting of 200 rad on each of 6 days was undertaken (Thomas 1982b). It was hoped that the fractionated regimen would decrease the likelihood of leukemic relapse following transplant and might be less toxic to the lungs. Fifty-three patients with ANL in first remission were entered into a randomized study. The longterm survival is 50% with a slightly better survival for the fractionated irradiation group.

Chronic myelogenous leukemia (CGL) is in fact not a chronic disease at all but indeed carries a very serious prognosis. Initially we undertook to transplant patients in blast crisis after failure of chemotherapy (Doney 1978). Of 12 such patients, only 1 had a remission beyond 1 year and he died at 16 months of recurrent leukemia. A second group of patients was conditioned with cyclophosphamide x 2 followed by fractionated irradiation, either 1200 rad or 1575 rad. Eight of 22 patients are alive and in remission from 4 to 48 months after grafting.

Since the median survival time for patients with the "chronic" phase of CGL is on the order of 2 to 4 years and there are no cures by conventional therapy, we began studies to treat this disease with marrow transplantation. Twelve patients who had cytogenetically normal identical twins to serve as marrow donors were given dimethylbusulfan, 5 mg/kg followed by cyclophosphamide and 1000 rad TBI (Fefer 1982). Eight of these patients are living, well and cytogenetically normal 24 to 68 months after transplantation. Encouraged by this apparent ability to eradicate the abnormal clone of leukemic cells we began a study of marrow grafting for patients with CGL in chronic phase who had an HLA identical sibling (Clift, in press). The patients are conditioned with 2 doses of cyclophosphamide followed by 200 rad irradiation on each of 6 days. They are then randomized to receive Methotrexate or cyclosporine for prevention of graft-versus-host disease. Thirteen patients have been entered on this study and 9 are living without the Philadelphia chromosome 5 to 20 months after grafting.

The major complications associated with marrow transplant are opportunistic infections, particularly viral complications, graft-versus-host disease and recurrence of leukemia. All of these complications are the subject of intensive research in Seattle and many other institutions. For example, efforts are now being made to take advantage of the graft-versus-leukemia effect by administration of additional donor buffy coat cells in the first 5 days after grafting (Weiden 1981). Buffy coat cells have been demonstrated to increase the incidence of chronic graft-versus-host disease. Since most cases of chronic GVHD are now treatable, it appears

worthwhile to attempt to utilize this method for inducing some additional chronic GVHD.

Cyclosporine is being used in a randomized trial
post grafting in comparison to the standard post
grafting Methotrexate regimen. Those studies will be
presented later during this meeting by Dr. Deeg.
Briefly, with 31 patients in each arm of the study,
there is no difference in survival with 70% of the
patients alive 1 year after grafting.

Since graft-versus-host disease is presumed to be
mediated by T cells, we and others are now attempting to
prevent graft-versus-host disease by in vitro treatment
of the donor marrow with monoclonal anti-T cell antibodies. In addition, these antibodies are being used in
vivo for treatment of established graft-versus-host
disease (Hansen 1981).

The administration of interferon postgrafting is
also being evaluated for its effect on the incidence and
severity of graft-versus-host disease, on the incidence
of viral interstitial pneumonias and on the incidence of
recurrence of leukemia. The Seattle Group is conducting
a prospective study randomizing patients to receive or
not to receive interferon in the first 80 days after
marrow grafting for patients with ALL in second remission. Although the study is still in progress, it
appears that cytomegalovirus interstitial pneumonia has
not been decreased but the incidence of recurrence of
leukemia is lower in patients given interferon. However, more patients and a longer period of followup are
necessary to complete this study.

One of the limiting factors for a potential marrow
graft recipient is the necessity of a normal marrow
donor. To extend the potential donor pool we have
undertaken marrow transplants using family member donors
who are 1 HLA haplotype genetically identical with the
patient and the other HLA haplotype phenotypically
identical at 2 of the 3 major loci (Clift 1979). More
than 80 such transplants have been carried out for
patients with leukemia and the results are similar to
those obtained for patients with HLA identical donors.
Patients with leukemia transplanted in relapse have a
long-term survival rate on the order of 20-30% while

those transplanted in remission have a long-term survival rate on the order of 50%. The incidence and severity of graft-versus-host disease has not been significantly different. In addition, the Seattle Team has carried out a transplant for ALL using a totally unrelated donor (Hansen 1980). The graft was successful without subsequent graft-versus-host disease, but the patient died of recurrent leukemia 18 months later. Several similar transplants have since been carried out at other centers. It is theoretically possible to form large panels of volunteer unrelated donors.

Up to the present, marrow grafting has been only occasionally employed in the treatment of other malignant diseases that might be expected to respond to high-dose chemoradiotherapy. The Seattle team transplanted 8 patients with advanced non-Hodgkin's lymphoma using identical twin donors (Appelbaum 1981). Eight are living in remission 2 to 12 years later. Eight of 20 similar patients given allogeneic grafts are in remission 3 to 57 months later.

In summary, patients under the age of 50 with acute leukemia and a suitable marrow donor now have the option of marrow grafting as an established treatment modality. For patients with ANL in first remission the results indicate 50-60% of these patients may be cured of their disease. For patients who have relapsed at least once, marrow grafting offers the possibility of a cure for approximately 20-30%. Marrow grafting is potentially applicable to patients with lymphoma, Hodgkin's disease, multiple myeloma, small cell lung cancer, testicular cancer and ovarian cancer. Studies to define the stage and type of tumor with a steep dose responsive curve to chemoradiotherapy are currently underway in many centers and the next few years should see a much broader application of marrow transplantation to the eradication of malignant disease.

REFERENCES

Appelbaum FR, Fefer A, Cheever MA, Buckner CD, Greenberg PD, Kaplan HG, Storb R, Thomas ED (1981). Treatment of non-Hodgkin's lymphoma with marrow transplantation in identical twins. Blood 58:509.

Buckner CD, Clift RA, Thomas ED, Sanders JE, Hackman R, Stewart PS, Storb R, Sullivan KM (1982a). Allogeneic marrow transplantation for patients with acute non-lymphoblastic leukemia in second remission. Leuk Res 6:395.

Buckner CD, Clift RA, Thomas ED, Sanders JE, Stewart PS, Storb R, Sullivan KM, Hackman R (1982b). Allogeneic marrow transplantation for acute non-lymphoblastic leukemia in relapse using fractionated total body irradiation. Leuk Res 6:389.

Clift RA, Hansen JA, Thomas ED, Buckner CD, Sanders JE, Mickelson EM, Storb R, Johnson FL, Singer JW, Goodell BW (1979). Marrow transplantation from donors other than HLA-identical siblings. Transplantation 28:235.

Clift RA, Buckner CD, Thomas ED, Sanders JE, Stewart PS, Sullivan KM, McGuffin R, Hersman J, Sale GE, Storb R (1982). Allogeneic marrow transplantation using fractionated total body irradiation in patients with acute lymphoblastic leukemia in relapse. Leuk Res 6:401.

Clift RA, Buckner CD, Thomas ED, Doney K, Fefer A, Neiman PE, Singer J, Sanders J, Stewart P, Sullivan KM, Deeg J, Storb R (In press). The treatment of chronic granulocytic leukemia in chronic phase by allogeneic marrow transplantation. Lancet.

Doney K, Buckner CD, Sale GE, Ramberg R, Boyd C, Thomas ED (1978). Treatment of chronic granulocytic leukemia by chemotherapy, total body irradiation and allogeneic bone marrow transplantation. Exp Hematol. 6:738-747, 1978.

Fefer A, Cheever MA, Thomas ED, Appelbaum FR, Buckner CD, Clift RA, Glucksberg H, Greenberg PD, Johnson FL, Kaplan HG, Sanders JE, Storb R, Weiden PL (1981). Bone marrow transplantation for refractory acute leukemia in 34 patients with identical twins. Blood 57:421.

Fefer A, Cheever MA, Greenberg PD, Appelbaum FR, Boyd CN, Buckner CD, Kaplan HG, Ramberg R, Sanders JE, Storb R, Thomas ED (1982). Treatment of chronic granulocytic leukemia with chemoradiotherapy and transplantation of marrow from identical twins. N Engl J Med 306:63.

Hansen JA, Clift RA, Thomas ED, Buckner CD, Storb R, Giblett ER (1980). Transplantation of marrow from an unrelated donor to a patient with acute leukemia. N Engl J Med 303:565.

Hansen JA, Martin PJ, Kamoun M, Torok-Storb B, Newman W, Nowinski RC, Thomas ED (1981). Monoclonal antibodies recognizing human T cells: Potential role for preventing graft-versus-host reactions following allogeneic marrow transplantation. Transplant Proc 13:1133.

Thomas ED, Storb R, Clift RA, Fefer A, Johnson FL, Neiman PE, Lerner KG, Glucksberg H, Buckner CD (1975). Bone-marrow transplantation. N Engl J Med 292:832,895.

Thomas ED, Ramberg RE, Sale GE, Sparkes RS, Golde DW (1976). Direct evidence for a bone marrow origin of the alveolar macrophage in man. Science 192:1016.

Thomas ED, Buckner CD, Banaji M, Clift RA, Fefer A, Flournoy N, Goodell BW, Hickman RO, Lerner KG, Neiman PE, Sale GE, Sanders JE, Singer J, Stevens M, Storb R, Weiden PL (1977). One hundred patients with acute leukemia treated by chemotherapy, total body irradiation, and allogeneic marrow transplantation. Blood 49:511.

Thomas ED, Clift RA, Buckner CD for the Seattle Marrow Transplant Team (1982a). Marrow transplantation for patients with acute nonlymphoblastic leukemia who achieve a first remission. Cancer Treat Rep, 66:1463.

Thomas ED, Clift RA, Hersman J, Sanders JE, Stewart P, Buckner CD, Fefer A, McGuffin R, Smith JW, Storb R (1982b). Marrow transplantation for acute nonlymphoblastic leukemia in first remission using fractionated or single-dose irradiation. Int J Rad Onc Biol Phys 8:817.

Weiden PL, Sullivan KM, Flournoy N, Storb R, Thomas ED, the Seattle Marrow Transplant Team (1981). Antileukemic effect of chronic graft-versus-host disease. Contribution to improved survival after allogeneic marrow transplantation. N Engl J Med 304:1529.

13th International Cancer Congress, Part A
Current Perspectives in Cancer, pages 141–143
© 1983 Alan R. Liss, Inc., 150 Fifth Avenue, New York, NY 10011

BIOLOGY AND ONCOLOGY: REGULATION OF GROWTH, DIFFERENTIATION
AND MALIGNANCY

Leo Sachs

Department of Genetics,
Weizmann Institute of Science,
Rehovot 76100, ISRAEL

Carcinogens and tumor promoters have pleiotropic effects.
Tumor initiators can induce a variety of genetic changes,
and tumor promoters can regulate a variety of physiological
molecules that control growth and differentiation. The
origin of malignancy involves a sequence of genetic changes,
including specific chromosome changes. After this sequence
of changes, some tumors can still be induced to revert with
a high frequency from a malignant to a non-malignant
phenotype. An understanding of the the mechanism that
controls growth and differentiation in normal cells would
seem to be an essential requirement to elucidate the
origin, evolution and reversibility of malignancy. In
illustrating this approach, I have mainly used examples
from our studies on normal and leukemic hematopoietic
cells.

The cloning and clonal differentiation of normal hematopoietic cells in culture has made it possible to study
the controls that regulate growth (multiplication) and
differentiation of normal hematopoietic cells and the
changes in these controls that occur in the origin and
evolution of leukemia. Experiments with normal hematopoietic precursors and their differentiation to specific
cell types have shown that normal cells require different
proteins for the induction of growth and for the induction
of differentiation. Identification of these normal regulators and the finding that the growth-inducing protein can
induce production of the differentiation-inducing protein,
have shown how growth and differentiation can be normally
coupled. The origin of malignancy involves uncoupling of
growth and differentiation, by changing the requirement for

growth without blocking cell response to the normal inducer
of differentiation. Addition of the normal differentiation-
inducing protein to these malignant cells can thus still
induce their normal differentiation. These differentiated
cells are then no longer malignant. This normal differentiation of leukemic cells has been obtained in vitro and in
vivo.

In some tumors, such as sarcomas, reversion from a
malignant to a non-malignant phenotype is due to segre-
gation of specific chromosomes from the malignant cells so
as to restore the normal growth control. However, in
myeloid leukemias, and presumably also in teratocarcinomas,
this reversion is due to induction of normal differentiation
in the malignant cells without correcting the genetic
abnormality that induces a change in the control of growth.
Genetic changes which produce blocks in the ability to be
induced to differentiate by the normal inducer can occur
later in the evolution of leukemia. But even these cells
may still be induced to differentiate by other compounds,
including low doses of compounds now being used in cancer
therapy, that can induce the differentiation program by
other pathways. Induction of normal differentiation in
malignant cells may therefore be of value as an approach to
cancer therapy.

The origin of leukemia appears to involve changes from an
inducible to a constitutive expression of genes that control
cell growth. These changes in gene expression can be produced by the integration of proviral sequences near growth
regulatory sites, or by specific chromosome changes that
produce differences in the balance of certain genes due to
changes in gene dosage. It seems that integration of proviral sequences has to be followed by the chromosome changes
for the cells to be malignant. Changes from inducible to
constitutive gene expression can produce asynchrony in the
co-ordination required for the normal developmental program.
Depending on the genes involved, this asynchrony then
produces the uncoupling of growth and differentiation and
the blocks in response to the normal differentiation-inducer
that occur in the origin and further evolution of malignancy.

Uncoupling of controls has been found in various types
of tumors. The above conclusions may thus be applicable to
malignancies derived from other types of cells, whose
normal growth and differentiation are controlled by other
physiological regulators. The existence of constitutive
expression of specific genes that uncouple controls in
malignant cells can also explain the expression of fetal

proteins and other specialized products of normal differentiation in various types of malignancies. The data discussed
in this lecture are reviewed in the references cited below.

REFERENCES

Sachs L (1974). Regulation of membrane changes, differentiation and malignancy in carcinogenesis. Harvey Lectures
68 New York: Academic Press pp 1-35.
Sachs L (1978). Control of normal cell differentiation and
the phenotypic reversion of malignancy in myeloid
leukemia. Nature 274:535-539.
Sachs L (1980). Constitutive uncoupling of pathways of
gene expression that control growth and differentiation
in myeloid leukemia: A model for the origin and progression of malignancy. Proc Natl Acad Sci USA 77:
6152-6156.
Sachs L (1982a). Control of growth and normal differentiation in leukemic cells. Regulation of the developmental
program and restoration of the normal phenotype in
myeloid leukemia. J Cell Physiol Suppl 1:151-164.
Sachs L (1982b). Normal developmental programmes in myeloid
leukemia. Regulatory proteins in the control of growth
and differentiation. Cancer Surveys 1 No. 2 Oxford
University Press pp 321-342.

13th International Cancer Congress, Part A
Current Perspectives in Cancer, pages 145–207
© **1983 Alan R. Liss, Inc., 150 Fifth Avenue, New York, NY 10011**

13TH INTERNATIONAL CANCER CONGRESS
SEATTLE, WASHINGTON, USA
SEPTEMBER 8-15, 1982

FINAL REPORT

Dr. Edwin A. Mirand, Secretary-General
Roswell Park Memorial Institute
666 Elm Street
Buffalo, NY 14263

TABLE OF CONTENTS

A) GENERAL REPORT - P. 1

        Background   148
        Scientific Program   150
        Publications   155
        Attendance   155
        Site   156
        Travel Coordinator   156
        Accommodations   157
        Transportation   157
        Communications   157
        Security   158
        Press Room   158
        Media Coverage   158
        Promotional Efforts   159
        Local Organizing Committee   161
        Social Program   161
        Volunteer Participation   162
        Opening Ceremony   163
        Closing Ceremony   164
        Staffing   164
        Funding Sources   165

B) ANALYSIS OF SCIENTIFIC PROGRAM - P. 166

        Daily Schedule   167
        National Program Committee Report   168
        Evaluation of Program Balance   191

C) COUNTRIES REPRESENTED AT THE CONGRESS - P. 192

D) PRESS ROOM REPORT - P. 193

E) SPECIAL MEETINGS AND FUNCTIONS - P. 194

F) EXHIBITS

        Commercial Exhibits   195
        Scientific Exhibits   197

G) OFFICE OF THE SECRETARIAT - P. 199

H) COMMITTEES OF THE CONGRESS - P. 200

National Organizing Committee   201
National Program Committee   203
International Science Committee   205
Officers   207
Board of Trustees   207

A. General Report

BACKGROUND

The 13th International Cancer Congress, sponsored by the
International Union Against Cancer, was held in Seattle,
Washington, USA, September 8th - 15th, 1982. More than
9,000 people participated in this quadrennial meeting
to exchange ideas about cancer research, treatment and
control. They came from 84 countries and their numbers
included physicians, scientists, nurses, allied health
professionals and volunteers. The host instutition for
the Congress was the Fred Hutchinson Cancer Research
Center.

On September 15, 1978 in Buenos Aires, Dr. William B.
Hutchinson, Director of the Fred Hutchinson Cancer
Research Center, and Dr. Edwin A. Mirand, Associate
Institute Director of Roswell Park Memorial Institute,
presented the proposal of the Fred Hutchinson Cancer
Research Center to host the 13th International Cancer
Congress in Seattle, Washington, USA. The proposal was
placed before the UICC Assembly and Council. The UICC
Assembly and Council after reviewing other proposals
from other countries, officially notified the USA
National Committee of the UICC of the acceptance of its
proposal by the Executive Director of the Geneva Office
of the UICC on November 29, 1978. On January 26, 1979
the USA National Committee of the UICC appointed the
officers of the Congress:

- Dr. William B. Hutchinson, President

- Dr. Edwin A. Mirand, Secretary-General

In addition, a National Organizing Committee, composed
of 21 members, with Dr. William B. Hutchinson as Chairman and Dr. Edwin A. Mirand as Co-Chairman was appointed
by the USA National Committee of the UICC in January,
1979. The Committee was representative of the various
cancer organization constituencies in the United States.
The first meeting of the National Organizing Committee
was held on June 28, 1979 at the Fred Hutchinson Cancer
Research Center in Seattle, Washington. At that meeting
the duties of the host country, as established by the
UICC, were outlined, and the Committee reviewed and
approved the appointments of Dr. Enrico Mihich as
Chairman of the National Program Committee and
Dr. Willis Taylor as Chairman of the Local Organizing
Committee. The site for the Congress meeting rooms and
facilities at the Seattle Center was inspected by the
National Organizing Committee. Dr. Hutchinson and
Dr. Mirand presented a tentative budget and organization
for the Congress which was approved, and English was
recommended as the official language of the Congress.

On July 30, 1979, after a site inspection of the Seattle
Center, the International Committee on Congresses of
the UICC agreed with the officers of the Congress and
the National Organizing Committee that the Center would
meet the needs of the 13th International Cancer Congress.
The Committee also approved the meeting schedule and
further agreed that English would be the official
language and there was no necessity to have simultaneous
translation in other languages.

In December 1980, in order to simplify the administration of the Congress and to reduce travel costs, the
USA National Committee of the UICC approved plans to
extablish a separate non-profit corporation to manage
and operate the 13th Congress. Thus the original
Articles of Incorporation and By-Laws were revised to
provide a five-member Board of Trustees responsible for
overseeing the affairs of the Congress. The Board
included both Dr. William Hutchinson, Dr. Edwin A.
Mirand, Dr. Stephen Carter, Mr. David Lycette, and

Mr. Francis J. Wilcox. Prior to the Congress, the Board met twice to review and approve Congress finances, contracts and activities.

SCIENTIFIC PROGRAM

Critical to the success of the 13th Congress was the National Program Committee, led by Dr. Enrico Mihich. The Committee met five times to finalize the Congress scientific program. The scientific program was approved by the Secretary-General upon thorough review by him. In selecting chairmen and co-chairmen, the Program Committee strived to adhere to the policy that each session would be led by an expert on the particular subject from a foreign country and co-chaired by a United States participant in order to promote the exchange of knowledge between countries.

Over 4,100 abstracts were received and reviewed by the National Program Committee and 4,087 were finally accepted for presentation. Over 775 invited presentations were made in plenary sessions, symposia, seminars, postgraduate courses, roundtable discussions, and the role of volunteer agencies in cancer control. The remaining papers were presented in proffered paper sessions, poster sessions, panels, and scientific films and exhibits. Commercial exhibits were also displayed.

Of the submitted presentations made at the Congress, 7.2% were panels, 29.3% were proffered papers, 62.3% were poster sessions, .7% were scientific films, and .5% were scientific exhibits. As many as 29 simultaneous sessions, representing 58 countries, were offered twice daily. To encourage interaction among program participants, there were ample opportunities for discussion.

An unusual emphasis distinguishing this Congress was the many nonphysicians participating in distinctive and formal programs specially designed for them. Although as a rule audiences attending this type of Congress are primarily physicians and scientists engaged in the field of oncology, great effort was made to provide formal programs for nurses, allied health personnel and people engaged in voluntary organizations such as the American

Cancer Society. For example, ten sessions on the role of voluntary groups in cancer control were conducted. These were planned in conjunction with the National Program Committee, the Secretary-General of the Congress and representatives from the American Cancer Society.

In establishing the scientific program of the Congress, it was agreed by the Committee and their consultants that major emphasis should be given to the following areas:

- The most significant advances in clinical investigations since the 12th International Cancer Congress.

- Progress in understanding the mechanisms of cell growth control and differentiation.

- Identification of biological responses that define tumor-host relationships.

- Development of new therapeutic approaches based on these advances.

- Progress in clarifying the mechanisms of chemical carcinogenesis and the genetic and environmental factors conditioning the development of cancer; and those factors related to socioeconomic and geographic influences.

- Subjects related to patient care and its organization, with particular emphasis on the indispensable functions of the professional nurse and the need for complex supportive structures that are essential in both the hospital and community setting for optimal delivery of care to cancer patients.

- Progress in managing most neoplastic diseases in humans was extensively reviewed. Examples include:

  - Advances in management of lymphomas, including improved diagnosis, classification and staging, including use of such approaches as monoclonal antibodies. Emphasis was given to the responses of this disease to combined modalities of treatment, particularly those involving radiotherapy, and the use of novel therapeutic approaches, including interferons.

- Progress in the management of malignant melanoma, particularly the use of surgical proceudres and results of chemoimmunotherapy. Problems in diagnosis, classification and prevention were also considered.

- Improvements in the management of breast cancer. Topics: the diagnosis and treatment of minimal breast cancer and the role of radiation treatments; progress in adjuvant chemotherapy and the definition of optimal surgical treatments; significance of therapy and the definition of optimal surgical treatments; significance of multidisciplinary approaches to the diagnosis of breast cancer, of the measurement of hormone receptors and of the assessment of the pathological features of the disease in the design of optimal treatments; value and limitations of screening for breast cancer; effects of dietary factors in breast carcinogenesis and the role of nutrition in the management of the disease; application of reconstructive surgery; and irradiation as a possible causative agent for breast cancer.

- Major advances recently made through use of bone marrow transplantation as an effective therapeutic approach towards the curative treatment of acute leukemias. These advances were discussed in terms of the current

state of the art, as well as its
future projections. Use of interferons in counteracting the limiting
complications of bone marrow transplantation therapies that are related
to viral infection was considered.

- Gastrointestinal neoplasias, including pancreatic and hepatic cancer.
Major efforts were directed toward
the identification of new treatments.
The state of the art in the management of these diseases was outlined.

- Advances in the management of lung
cancer were discussed from a multidisciplinary point of view. Improvements in the pathological identification of incipient neoplasia and in
the assessment of pathological
determinants of prognosis were considered. Smoking and other etiological factors were assessed.

- Several other types of neoplasia
were considered, in most cases from
a multidisciplinary point of view;
and the state of the art was reviewed
with emphasis on the special requirements related to the characteristics
of these diseases and to the difficulties that need to be overcome
toward their definitive management.

- Areas where progress has been matched
by controversy are those related to
the design and evaluation of clinical
trials, and to the classification
and staging of various neoplastic
diseases. Selected topics in these
areas were extensively discussed.

- Major advances in radiotherapy were
reviewed particularly as related to
the use of high LET particles, the
development of effective radiation

oncology, and the therapeutic potential of photoirradiation and hyperthermia.

- Information on the possibility of
  effecting both cancer causation and
  therapy through dietary manipulations
  was discussed in depth.

- The increasing role of dentistry as
  an oncological specialty dealing
  with the management of neoplasias of
  the oral cavity was outlined and
  selective topics reviewed.

- Epidemiology of cancer, with emphasis
  on those aspects that are related to
  geographical, environmental and occupational influences on carcinogenesis
  and the genetic and hormonal factors
  affecting this process, were presented.

- The functions and impact of the
  oncology nurse in different parts of
  the world were discussed with emphasis on clinical research.

- The integration of diversified
  approaches to patient care in the
  hospice, the socioeconomic aspects
  involved in the care of the cancer
  patient, the team approach to rehabilitation, the psychosocial impact
  of cancer and the supportive
  structures of community care versus
  the role of cancer centers were all
  discussed in an effort to give
  attention to the need for a broad
  set of approaches focused on the
  optimal management of cancer.

In addition, 11 plenary lectures were offered twice
daily in the Seattle Center Arena, featuring topics
such as advances in cancer therapeutics; environmental
mutagens, carcinogens and tumor promoters; the role of

volunteer agencies; epidemiology and advances in cancer therapeutics.

Described as a well-balanced program, scientific
sessions were scheduled daily except Sunday, from
0830-1100 and from 1500-1730 with plenary lectures
beginning on September 10th from 1115-1215 and from
1345-1445. Last-minute cancellations and "no-shows"
were minimal. An additional plenary lecture was
scheduled on September 10th at 1245, and two special
evening sessions were provided. Daily schedule highlights were printed in a Congress newspaper, published
four times during the week of the Congress.

PUBLICATIONS

The program and the Proceedings containing abstracts
were published by Waverly Press, Inc. and distributed
to Congress delegates. Its 715 pages cover 4,087
abstracts. Extra copies of the Proceedings may be
purchased for $25 each. The archival volumes of the
13th International Cancer Congress will be published
by Alan R. Liss Publishers, Inc. They will include
the presentations made in the plenary Congress
lectures and the Congress symposia in a series of
volumes, arranged by subject area.

Audiotaping of Congress lectures, general symposia,
post-graduate courses, seminars, roundtable discussions, and sessions on the role of volunteer societies
and leagues in cancer control was provided by Audio-
Stats, Inc. The tapes were sold during the Congress
and made available for sale after the Congress.

ATTENDANCE

Using similar attendance categories as those established
at the 10th International Cancer Congress in Houston,
statistics of attendance indicate significant increases
in several categories, including those registering
as members, press, commercial exhibitors and volunteers.

13th INTERNATIONAL CANCER CONGRESS - ATTENDANCE

```
                        MEMBER REGISTRANTS:   5,390
                 SOCIAL MEMBER REGISTRANTS:     684
                STUDENT MEMBER REGISTRANTS:     211


  Other Registrants:


                                    Press:     150
            Commercial Exhibitors and Staff:   1,075
                  Secretarial and Officials:     150
          Volunteers, Hostesses and Local
                     Organizing Committee:    1,341

                              GRAND TOTAL:    9,001*
```

*This figure does not include those who participated in special meetings and functions associated with the Congress, such as the President's Cancer Panel and numerous cancer organizations.

SITE

The site of the 13th Congress was the 75-acre Seattle Center, location of the World's Fair in 1962. Most of the Center's meeting space was utilized by the Congress. The Center's largest facility, the Coliseum, housed poster sessions, scientific exhibits, ticket sales and registration activities. The 110 commercial exhibits, managed by Steven K. Herlitz, Inc., administrative offices, post office and message center were located in the 40,000 square foot Exhibition Hall. UICC Meetings held from September 5-18, 1982 were held at the Westin Hotel. The UICC officers and staff were very pleased with the accommodations.

OFFICIAL TRAVEL COORDINATOR

Accommodations, travel arrangements, tours and airport welcoming for the Cancer Congress delegates were coordinated by Princess Tours of Seattle, Washington, the

official travel coordinator for the 13th Congress.
Princess Tours also provided a computerized registration system for the Congress.

ACCOMMODATIONS

Prior to the Congress, over 6,000 rooms were reserved
in every major hotel and motel in Greater Seattle. As
the Congress approached, a few of the rooms not needed,
particularly those in the far outlying areas, were
released back to the hotels. Housing was booked through
Princess Tours on a first-come, first-served basis,
beginning with the downtown business district which
accommodated the majority of delegates.

For late registrants and those on limited budgets,
rooms at the University of Washington were available.
An accurate tally of the total number of rooms used by
Congress delegates is difficult to determine, since
some registrants made their own accommodation reservations outside the official travel coordinator, and
others changed hotels during the Congress. However,
Princess Tours estimates that at least 4,615 rooms
were used and 46 hotels booked through their office.
Major arrival dates were September 7th and 8th; major
departure dates were September 15th and 16th.

TRANSPORTATION

Transportation between hotels in the downtown area and
the Seattle Center was available to delegates free of
charge on the Monorail. Delegates in other areas
relied upon a shuttlebus service coordinated by
Princess Tours and Evergreen Trailways. During peak
hour service, over 43 buses were utilized; mid-day
shuttle service used fewer buses. Buses were also
available to all daytime special and cultural events
and for special evening cultural functions.

COMMUNICATIONS

Pacific Northwest Bell installed phones in each meeting
room at the Seattle Center, utilizing the City's

Centrex system for internal calls. Outside lines were
installed throughout the center including the Press
Room, volunteer and administrative offices and all
service areas.

SECURITY

Security at the Seattle Center was coordinated by the
Seattle Police Department and Seattle Center personnel,
using off-duty police for around-the-clock extra
security in the Exhibition Hall and Coliseum. Due to
the number of buses in peak traffic hours, special
security officers were hired to direct traffic flow
around the Seattle Center.

PRESS ROOM

Over 150 writers, photographers and television reporters from the USA and a variety of other countries
attended the Congress. The Press Room operated from
September 7th through September 15th, except
September 12th, from 7:30 a.m. to as late as 8:00 or
9:00 p.m., with a paid staff of seven and several
professional volunteers.

Prior to the Congress, three general mailings were
made to media people, including regional, national and
international science and medical writers, columnists
and editors of appropriate medical periodicals.

The Press Room featured a general working area for the
press and a room for press conferences and briefings.
The Press Room was well equipped with typewriters,
telex and telecopiers, telephones and copy machines.

MEDIA COVERAGE

This Congress undoubtedly received far more television
coverage - local, national and international - than
any previous Congress. Though there was some early
discussion on the possibility of transmitting the more
important programs by satellite to UICC member countries
around the world, this did not come to pass because of

the excessive cost. The major American television and
radio networks were advised, along with other media, of
plans for the Congress. Later, Cable News Network and
the new Cable Health Network were invited. National
coverage of the Congress was done by NBC, whose Frank
Field scheduled and filmed a series of interviews
and features, also for later broadcast. Alan Landsburg
Productions filmed a documentary, presumably for sale
to networks or individual stations, as did Armand
Hammer Productions. National Public Radio sent a
reporter. Similarly, overseas television networks
were invited to attend. A local film crew was hired
by Mucio Athayde to film presentation of the Athayde
award for use by Brazilian television. Television
and radio coverage also came from Yorkshire Television
in Leeds, England; Niikei-McGraw-Hill, Incorporated,
Tokyo, Japan; Swedish Broadcasting Corporation;
Radio-TV Luxembourg; and ANB Television, Tokyo, which
sent a crew from Japan with an American coordinator.

Local radio and television stations were thoroughly
briefed prior to the Congress and coverage was
extensive. In addition to daily news coverage of
Congress events and personalities by all prinicpal
stations, many features were filmed. For instance,
Station KOMO-TV, the Seattle ABC affiliate, developed
eight features on cancer incidence, head and neck
cancer, leukemia developments, lung cancer developments,
cancer patients overcoming odds, and cancer and diet,
in addition to numerous interviews. Though stations
KING-TV and KIRO-TV filmed fewer stories, each did
several interviews or features, and did Viacom
Cablevision.

PROMOTIONAL EFFORTS

In addition to invitations to the media, several comprehensive efforts were made prior to the Congress to
draw delegates. Eighty thousand (80,000) "first
circulars" announcing the meeting were mailed worldwide to all national and international cancer
institutes and to all national and international
cancer societies. In April 1980, 85,000 "Congress
Updates" were distributed, and more than 150,000
people received copies of the "Advance Program

Announcement," which contained information concerning Congress registration, the submission of abstracts, accommodations, tours and a preliminary outline of the Congress scientific program. This was followed up by another brochure mailed to 35,000 in the United States describing both the scientific and social program schedule and including forms for advance ticket orders. Special mailings were also sent to state medical associations in the Pacific Northwest. Further, personal efforts were made by Dr. Mirand, who attended medical conferences throughout the world to promote the 13th Congress. This effort took the Secretary-General to Europe - Norway, Switzerland, France, South America - Brazil, the Orient - Japan, and throughout the United States at various cancer meetings. Announcements about the Congress were also published in numerous biomedical newspapers and many journals. Cancer Research featured a special journal cover on its May 1982 issue.

A list below provides some of the journals in which the Congress was highlighted. They are as follows:

Cancer News
Cancer Research (5/82 - Cover)
Ca-A Cancer Journal for Clinicians (7/81 - Cover)
Cancer Letter
ARAB Medical Journal
Oncology Times
ACR Bulletin
Bulletin, American College of Surgeons
EORTC Newsletter (Switzerland)
National Newsletter - Canadian Cancer Society
Organization of European Cancer Institutes (12/81)
Journal of the American Medical Association
University of Washington Medical Bulletin
Research Resources Reports
U.S. and International Dental Journals
News release sent to Science/Medical Writers and
   Medical Journal Editors - National and International
Society of Surgical Oncology News
Medi Congress (Brussels)
Journal of Western Medicine
NCI - Nutrition and Cancer
Medizinsche Kangresse '82 (Baden, Germany)
Cancer Forum (Australia)

ACCC Newsletter
American Society of Cell Biology Newsletter
American Association of Immunologists
Medical Meetings
Fred Hutchinson Cancer Research Newsletter Special
  Issue 1982
RPMI Clinical Newsletters (1979-1982)
UICC Bulletin (6/80, 10/80, 11/81, 12/81, Vol 19 #2
  July 1982)
Associated Organizations of International Interests
  (7/82, 8/82, 9/82)
Travel Host (September 5, 1982)

LOCAL ORGANIZING COMMITTEE

The Local Organizing Committee, led by Dr. Willis
Taylor, Chairman, and greatly assisted by Dr. James
Wilson, Co-Chairman, met weekly for two and a half
years, making local arrangements and coordinating the
activities of the twelve subcommittees which were:

        Airport Welcoming - T. Evans Wycoff, Chairman
        Emergency Care - Bruce Stevenson, M.D., Chairman
        Exhibits - Ward Wren, Chairman
        Foreign Hospitality - Gordon Clinton, Chairman
        Housing - Bob Hannah, Chairman
        Local Finance - Hunter Simpson, Chairman
        Public Relations - Mark Cooper, Chairman
        Scientific Tours - John Dawson, M.D.
        Social Affairs - Mary Martin and Wilma Maurel,
          Co-Chairwomen
        Special Services - Bob Arnold, Chairman
        Transportation - Sam Sherer, Chairman
        Volunteers Staffing - Betsy Pommerening,
          Chairwoman

SOCIAL PROGRAM

The Secretary-General of the Congress authorized the
Local Organizing Committee much latitude in developing
the social program and was extremely helpful in the
development. For instance, the Committee planned for
one main social or cultural function each day and
evening during the Congress, with each day's program

of activities scheduled to accommodate 2,500 to 3,000 delegates. Where economically possible, free events were offered to delegates on a first-come, first-served basis. Other events required an average payment of $10-$15 each, including refreshments. The local program was developed, based on the response to a questionnaire printed on the back of the Congress registration form.

Daytime events included tours of a Boeing airplane factory; a shopping tour; coffee hours at the Governor's Mansion and the University of Washington; private club luncheons; tours and teas at local museums; a garden tour; and a tour of the only school in the United States devoted to glass art.

Evening entertainment sponsored by the Local Organizing Committee for Congress delegates consisted of a performance by the Seattle Symphony Orchestra; a concert by the Philadelphia String Quartet; wine-tasting and salmon dinners at Chateau Ste. Michelle; an evening of jazz; and two evenings of entertainment featuring the Pacific Northwest Ballet.

As expected the free events were most popular, but non-free events were not as well attended as anticipated. This may be explained by the fact that official receptions and evening seminars were often in direct competition with evening cultural events. Also, the high cost of attending the Congress might have had some impact on these optional events.

VOLUNTEER PARTICIPATION

Each of the 25 events sponsored by the Local Organizing Committee was coordinated by a volunteer subcommittee of the Social Affairs Committee. As noted in the Congress attendance figures, volunteer participation in the 13th Congress was high. In addition to those who organized the local social and cultural program, during the Congress alone 856 positions were filled by volunteers who contributed an estimated 4,376 hours serving as information clerks, session aides, messengers, office assistants, registration aides and press room attendants. The response of the Seattle community

to the Congress needs was greatly appreciated, particularly by the Secretariat since this helped to keep
Congress expenditures down. Volunteers also stuffed
more than 10,000 delegate bags prior to the Congress.
Every volunteer received a written job description and
all volunteers either attended an orientation meeting
or received training materials. Recognizing the important contrubution made by volunteers to the success of
the 13th Congress, Dr. Mirand hosted a reception in
their honor on the evening of September 14th at the
Four Seasons Olympic Hotel.

OPENING CEREMONY

Volunteers were also instrumental in planning the
Opening Ceremony of the 13th International Cancer
Congress, which was held on Thursday, September 9th
at 6:00 p.m. in the Seattle Center Arena. Drawing
an estimated 5,500, the Opening Ceremony was one of
the best-attended events of the Congress. The Master
of Ceremonies was Mr. T.A. Wilson, Chairman of the
Board of the Boeing Company. Welcoming remarks were
given by Dr. Umberto Veronesi, UICC President;
Dr. Edwin A. Mirand, Secretary-General of the Congress;
and the Honorable Charles Royer, Mayor of the City of
Seattle. Governor John Spellman of the State of
Washington gave the keynote address, commending
delegates for their role as pioneers of mankind in the
field of science.

The Secretariat was disappointed at the absence of
President Reagan   Vice President Bush. However,
President Reagan sent a representative to the Congress,
National Cancer Institute Director, Dr. Vincent DeVita,
who read the President's message at the Opening
Ceremony.

A highlight of the Opening Ceremony was the presentation
of the Mucio Athyade Prize, a $100,000 prize awarded to
Dr. Charles Heidelberger by the Mucio Athayde Foundation
of Brazil. As Dr. Heidelberger was not able to attend
due to illness, his wife accepted the award on his
behalf.

Throughout the evening, entertainment interludes were
provided by the Fort Lewis Army Band, the Northwest
Boy's Choir and the Seattle Symphony Brass Ensamble.
Following the ceremony, a complimentary reception
featuring Washington State wines and domestic cheeses
was held in the Seattle Center Opera House, which was
superbly decorated by members of the Seattle Garden
Club under the direction of Mrs. Doyle Fowler.

CLOSING CEREMONY

The Closing Ceremony was held on September 15th at
6:00 p.m. in the Seattle Center Opera House.
Dr. William B. Hutchinson, Congress President and
Dr. Antonio Junqueira, President of the UICC, made
important remarks to the audience and Dr. Gerald P.
Murphy, UICC Secretary-General, presented honors and
awards on behalf of the UICC, particularly to
Dr. Hutchinson and Dr. Mirand for their efforts with
the Congress. Entertainment was provided by the Air
Force Band of the Pacific Northwest and the Island
City Jazz Band.

STAFFING

Established more than three and a half years prior to
the Congress, the organization of the 13th International
Cancer Congress in Seattle consisted of three full-time
employees, and three part-time consultants. The full-
time members included an operations manager responsible
for monitoring Congress finances, a director of services
who coordinated local planning and arrangements, and an
administrative assistant. The consultants advised the
Secretary-General on public relations, publications
and other administrative matters. In addition to the
Seattle staff, most all of the Secretariat activities
of the Congress were conducted by the Secretary-General
at Roswell Park Memorial Institute in Buffalo, where a
staff of up to 25 people developed the scientific
program and promotion of the Congress. Less than three

months prior to the Congress the Seattle staff more than doubled, and during the week of the meeting the staff, including paid temporary help, increased to sixty employees.

FUNDING SOURCES

Major funding sources for the 13th International Cancer Congress were the National Cancer Institute, the National and local American Cancer Society, and the Pacific Northwest Regional Commission. Registration fees made up 50.53% of the total Congress budget, which was approximately $1,458,178. Other sources of funds and in kind contributions were: Roswell Park Memorial Institute, Fred Hutchinson Cancer Research Center, Abbott Laboratories, the Boeing Company, Ciba Pharmaceuticals, the City of Seattle, Lederle Laboratories, Mead Johnson Pharmaceutical Division, Pan American Airlines, Parke Davis, Princess Tours, Rainer National Bank, Safeco Inc., Stuart Pharmaceuticals, Swedish Hospital, United Airlines and The Upjohn Company. The Washington State Division of the American Cancer Society underwrote the delegate portfolios; G.M. Nameplate prepared the brass key tags; Liberty Orchards provided "aplets and cotlets" candy; and the Washington State Department of Commerce and Economic Development supplied brochures. In addition the Greater Seattle Fuschia Society, Job's Daughters, Pacific Fruit and Produce, Parkwood Services, the Puget Sound Dahlia Association, the Seattle Chrysanthemum Society, the Seattle Rose Society and the Washington State Apple Commission contributed to the Congress Opening and Closing Ceremonies.

B.   Analysis of Scientific Program

SUMMARY

The program of the 13th International Cancer Congress
consisted of 9 general symposia, 48 symposia, 20 post-
graduate courses, 21 seminars, 31 roundtables, 30 panels,
99 proffered paper sessions, 89 poster sessions, 10
sessions on the role of volunteer societies, 22 films,
2 special sessions and 11 plenary lectures.

SCIENTIFIC PROGRAM

Summary:

Sept.8 A	Sept.9 M	Sept.9 A	Sept.10 M	Sept.10 A	Sept.11 M	Sept.11 A	Sept.13 M	Sept.13 A	Sept.14 M	Sept.14 A	Sept.15 M	Sept.15 A
GS-1	GS-4	GS-7	CS-1	CS-6	CS-10	CS-15	CS-19	CS-24	CS-28	CS-33	CS-37	CS-42
GS-2	GS-5	GS-8	CS-2	CS-7	CS-11	CS-16	CS-20	CS-25	CS-29	CS-34	CS-38	CS-43
GS-3	GS-4	GS-9	CS-3	CS-8	CS-12	CS-17	CS-21	CS-26	CS-30	CS-35	CS-39	CS-44
			CS-4	CS-9	CS-13	CS-18	CS-22	PGC-11	CS-31	CS-36	CS-40	CS-45
			CS-5	PGC-3	CS-14	PGC-7	CS-23	CS-27	CS-32	PGC-15	CS-41	CS-46
			PGC-1	PGC-4	PGC-5	PGC-8	PGC-9	PGC-12	PGC-13	PGC-16	PGC-17	CS-47
			PGC-2	P-4	PGC-4	P-10	PGC-10	P-16	PGC-14	P-21	PGC-18	CS-48
			P-1	P-5	P-7	P-11	P-13	P-17	P-18	P-22	P-24	PGC-19
			RVS-1	RVS-2	RVS-3	RVS-4	RVS-5	RVS-6	RVS-7	RVS-8	RVS-9	RVS-10
			SEM-1	SEM-3	SEM-5	SEM-7	SEM-9	SEM-11	SEM-13	SEM-15	SEM-18	SEM-20
			SEM-2	SEM-4	SEM-6	SEM-8	SEM-10	SEM-12	SEM-14	SEM-16	SEM-19	SEM-21
			P-2	P-6	P-8	P-12	P-14		P-19	SEM-17	P-25	PGC-20
			P-3	RT-4	P-9	RT-11	P-15	RT-18	P-20	P-23	P-26	P-27
			RT-1	RT-5	RT-8	RT-12	RT-15	RT-19	RT-22	RT-25	RT-28	P-28
			RT-2	RT-6	RT-9	RT-13	RT-16	RT-20	RT-23	RT-26	RT-29	P-29
			RT-3	RT-7	RT-10	RT-14	RT-17	RT-21	RT-24	RT-27	RT-30	RT-31
			PPS-1	PPS-11	PPS-21	PPS-31	PPS-41	PPS-51	PPS-61	PPS-71	PPS-81	P-30
			PPS-2	PPS-12	PPS-22	PPS-32	PPS-42	PPS-52	PPS-62	PPS-72	PPS-82	PPS-91
			PPS-3	PPS-13	PPS-23	PPS-33	PPS-43	PPS-53	PPS-63	PPS-73	PPS-83	PPS-92
			PPS-4	PPS-14	PPS-24	PPS-34	PPS-44	PPS-54	PPS-64	PPS-74	PPS-84	PPS-93
			PPS-5	PPS-15	PPS-25	PPS-35	PPS-45	PPS-55	PPS-65	PPS-75	PPS-85	PPS-94
			PPS-6	PPS-16	PPS-26	PPS-36	PPS-46	PPS-56	PPS-66	PPS-76	PPS-86	PPS-95
			PPS-7	PPS-17	PPS-27	PPS-37	PPS-47	PPS-57	PPS-67	PPS-77	PPS-87	PPS-96
			PPS-8	PPS-18	PPS-28	PPS-38	PPS-48	PPS-58	PPS-68	PPS-78	PPS-88	PPS-97
			PPS-9	PPS-19	PPS-29	PPS-39	PPS-49	PPS-59	PPS-69	PPS-79	PPS-89	PPS-98
			PPS-10	PPS-20	PPS-30	PPS-40	PPS-50	PPS-60	PPS-70	PPS-80	PPS-90	PPS-99
			PS1-9	PS10-18	PS19-27	PS28-36	PS37-45	PS46-53	PS54-62	PS63-71	PS72-80	PS81-89
			SE	SE	SE	SE	SE	SE	SE	SE	SE	SE
			SFS-1	SFS-2	SFS-3	SFS-4	SFS-5	SFS-6	SFS-7	SFS-8	SFS-9	

Legend:
PCL: Plenary Congress Lectures
GS : General Symposia
CS : Congress Symposia
PGC: Post-Graduate Courses
P : Panels
RVS: Role of Volunteer Societies & Leagues in Cancer Control
SEM: Seminars
PPS: Proffered Paper Sessions
PS : Poster Sessions
SFS: Scientific Sessions
SE : Scientific Exhibits

13th INTERNATIONAL CANCER CONGRESS

A Report Submitted on Behalf of the

National Program Committee

by

Enrico Mihich, M. D., Chairman

and

Judith S. Felski, Assistant

October 29, 1982

NATIONAL PROGRAM COMMITTEE REPORT

Summary:

The NPC Report comprises 8 tables reflecting:

       I)   Invited sessions - breakdown by country
      II)   Abstract rejections
     III)   Submitted sessions - breakdown by country
      IV)   Submitted sessions - total presentations of
            country be event (%)
       V)   Submitted sessions - percentage event total by
            country
      VI)   Individuals who met the commitment of a scheduled
            paper
     VII)   Cancellations/Replacements after May 1, 1982
            (invited sessions)
    VIII)   Evaluation: Comments solicited from Session
            Chairpersons

Table 1 is a breakdown by country of the Congress events by invitation. This tabulation also includes figures for chairpersons for the panel and proffered paper sessions. There were 47 countries represented in the sessions by invitation. US representation was 284/755.

Table II indicates the number of abstracts found not worthy of inclusion in the program, which was set up at a meeting of the National Program Committee in March 1982. A total of 39 abstracts from 15 countries were rejected.

Table III is a breakdown by country of the submitted Congress events (panel, proffered paper, poster, film and scientific exhibit sessions). There was a total of 3,312 presentations representing 58 countries. Of this overall total, 7.2% were panel presentations, 29.3% were proffered paper presentations, and 62.3% were poster presentations.

Table IV shows the number of presentations of each country broken down into event, and the % by event of that country's total.

Table V shows the % of each event total presented by the 58 participating countries.

Table VI represents statistics of individuals meeting the commitment of a scheduled presentation. The figure of 89.1% who met their commitment was based on the following: Of 1208 scheduled panel and proffered paper presentations, 67 individuals informed the National Program Committee office prior to the Congress of their inability to be present. A figure of 64 no shows was determined as a result of reviewing the post-session report submitted by the session chairperson. It is pointed out that statistics could not be determined for the poster, film or exhibit sessions as there was no appointed chairperson of these events. Also, not all chairperson reports were returned completed to the program Committee Office (115/128 or 89.8% were returned).

Table VII reflects the activity from May 1, 1982 in replacing chairpersons or speakers of the sessions by invitation. A total replacement of 90/1159 indicates that 7.8% of the invited program, plus chairpersons of the panel and proffered paper sessions, underwent replacement within the last four months prior to the Congress.

Table VIII is a listing of comments extracted from the post-session reports submitted by the session chairperson. It is again to be noted that not all reports were completed or returned to the Program Committee office.

Changes Made During the Congress: Although it is not possible to indicate specifics, the estimate of the changes made during the time of the Congress is 25 and included situations such as the following: (1) In several instances when a replacement was needed during an invited session, a local person was contacted to do this; (2) There were a number of cases where presentations originally scheduled as posters were, at the request of the author and due to the fact that the final scheduling card was not received (probably due to postal problems), used to fill in where there were known openings in the panel or proffered paper sessions of the program; (3) In several instances replacement of chairpersons needed to be accomplished, usually from within the session itself.

Respectfully submitted,

Enrico Mihich, M. D., Chairman
National Program Committee

Judith S. Felski, Program
Committee Assistant

10/29/82

TABLE 1

INVITED SESSIONS - FINAL BREAKDOWN BY COUNTRY
(includes Chairpersons of Panels/Proffered Papers and Two
Special Seminars)

Argentina	7
Australia	20
Austria	3
Belgium	6
Brazil	1
Canada	40
Chile	3
China	9
Colombia	1
Czechoslovakia	3
Denmark	8
Egypt	4
Fed. Rep. of Germany	34
Finland	4
France	38
German Dem. Rep.	4
Greece	3
Hong Kong	2
Hungary	13
India	3
Ireland	2
Israel	16
Italy	45
Japan	47
Kuwait	1
Netherlands	18
New Zealand	1
Nigeria	2
Norway	7
Pakistan	1
Paraguay	1
Peru	2
Poland	3
Rep. of Panama	1
Singapore	3
South Africa	4
Spain	3
Sweden	34

TABLE 1 (Continued)

Switzerland	13
Thailand	3
Tunisia	1
United Kingdom	61
United States	284
USSR	9
Uruguay	1
Venezuela	3
Yugoslavia	3
Total	775

TABLE II

ABSTRACT REJECTIONS RESULTING FROM
NATIONAL PROGRAM COMMITTEE MEETING - MARCH, 1982

Australia	1
Canada	1
Chile	1
China	1
Denmark	1
Fed. Rep. of Germany	2
France	1
Italy	7
Japan	5
Paraguay	1
Peru	3
Philippines	1
United States	11
United Kingdom	1
Yugoslavia	2
Total	39

TABLE III

SUBMITTED SESSIONS: BREAKDOWN BY COUNTRY

Country	Panel	Proffered Paper	Poster	Film	Exhibit	Total
Algeria			2			2
Argentina	2	12	60	1		75
Australia	3	5	12			20
Austria	2	5	8	2		17
Belgium	1	1	9			11
Brazil		5	8			13
Bulgaria	1	1	1			3
Cameroon			1			1
Canada	2	22	33	2		59
Chile			2			2
China		12	17			29
Colombia			6			6
Cuba		1	2			3
Czechoslovakia			1			1
Denmark	1	7	9			17
Egypt		7	13			20
Fed. Rep. of Germany	8	49	97			154
Finland	2	5	13			20
France	11	38	83	2	1	135
German Dem Rep		1	1			2
Greece		3	6			9
Hungary	1	4	6			11
India	1	15	61	6		83
Indonesia		1	4			5
Iran			1			1
Iraq			2			2
Ireland			2			2
Israel	2	9	26			37
Italy	9	69	202	2	1	283
Japan	24	151	341	1	1	518
Korea			3			3
Kuwait	1		1			2
Lebanon			1			1
Liberia			1			1
Mexico			2			2
Netherlands	4	9	8			21

TABLE III (Continued)

Country	Panel	Proffered Paper	Poster	Film	Exhibit	Total
New Zealand		2	5			7
Nigeria	1		6			7
Norway	3	11	23			37
Paraguay		1	2			3
Peru			2			2
Poland			7			7
Portugal			2			2
Rumania		4	17			21
Saudi Arabia		2	7			9
South Africa	1	4	9			14
Spain		8	19	3		30
Sweden	4	32	47			83
Switzerland	3	8	11	1		23
Tanzania			1			1
Thailand	1					1
Tunisia			2			2
Uganda		1				1
United Kingdom	11	19	38			68
United States	135	441	786	2	14	1378
USSR	2	2	16			20
Venezuela		1	1			2
Yugoslavia	1	3	19			23
Total	237	971	2065	22	17	3312
% Total	7.2	29.3	62.3	.7	.5	

The above figures are based on known cancellations in the program.

TABLE IV

SUBMITTED SESSIONS: TOTAL PRESENTATIONS
OF COUNTRY BY EVENT (%)

Country	Panel	Proffered Paper	Poster	Film	Exhibit	Total
Algeria			100.0			2
Argentina	2.6	16.0	80.0	1.3		75
Australia	15.0	25.0	60.0			20
Austria	11.8	29.4	47.0	11.8		17
Belgium	9.0	9.0	81.8			11
Brazil		38.5	61.5			13
Bulgaria	33.3	33.3	33.3			3
Cameroon			100.0			1
Canada	3.3	37.3	55.9	3.5		59
Chile			100.0			2
China		41.4	58.6			29
Colombia			100.0			6
Cuba		33.3	66.7			3
Czechoslovakia			100.0			1
Denmark	5.9	41.2	52.9			17
Egypt		35.0	65.0			20
Fed. Rep. of Germany	5.2	31.8	63.0			154
Finland	10.0	25.0	65.0			20
France	8.1	28.1	61.5	1.5	0.8	135
German Dem. Rep.		50.0	50.0			2
Greece		33.3	66.7			9
Hungary	9.0	36.4	54.6			11
India	1.2	18.1	73.5	7.2		83
Indonesia		20.0	80.0			5
Iran			100.0			1
Iraq			100.0			2
Ireland			100.0			2
Israel	5.4	24.3	70.3			37
Italy	3.2	24.4	71.4	0.7	0.3	283
Japan	4.6	29.1	65.9	0.2	0.2	518
Korea			100.0			3
Kuwait	50.0		50.0			2
Lebanon			100.0			1
Liberia			100.0			1

TABLE IV (Continued)

Country	Panel	Proffered Paper	Poster	Film	Exhibit	Total
Mexico			100.0			2
Netherlands	19.0	43.0	38.0			21
New Zealand		28.6	71.4			7
Nigeria	14.3		85.7			7
Norway	8.0	29.8	62.2			37
Paraguay		33.3	66.7			3
Peru			100.0			2
Poland			100.0			7
Portugal			100.0			2
Rumania		19.0	81.0			21
Saudi Arabia		22.2	77.8			9
South Africa	7.1	28.6	64.3			14
Spain		26.7	63.3	10.0		30
Sweden	4.8	38.6	56.6			83
Switzerland	13.0	34.8	47.8	4.4		23
Tanzania			100.0			1
Thailand	100.0					1
Tunisia			100.0			2
Uganda		100.0				1
United Kingdom	16.2	27.9	55.9			68
United States	9.8	32.0	57.0	0.1	1.1	1378
USSR	10.0	10.0	80.0			20
Venezuela		50.0	50.0			2
Yugoslavia	4.3	13.1	82.6			23

TABLE V

SUBMITTED SESSIONS: % EVENT TOTAL

Country	Panel (237)	Proffered Paper (971)	Poster (2065)	Film (22)	Exhibit (17)	Over-all (3312)
Algeria			.09			.06
Argentina	.80	1.24	2.90	4.54		2.26
Australia	1.30	.50	.58			.60
Austria	.80	.50	.40	9.09		.51
Belgium	.40	.10	.44			.33
Brazil		.50	.40			.39
Bulgaria	.40	.10	.04			.09
Cameroom	.80		.04			.03
Canada		2.27	1.60	9.09		1.78
Chile			.09			.06
China		1.24	.82			.88
Colombia			.29			.18
Cuba		.10	.09			.09
Czechoslovakia			.04			.03
Denmark	.40	.70	.44			.51
Egypt		.70	.63			.60
Fed. Rep. of Germany	3.40	5.01	4.70			4.65
Finland	.80	.50	.63		5.88	.60
France	4.60	3.91	4.02	9.09		4.08
German Dem. Rep.		.10	.04			.06
Greece		.30	.29			.27
Hungary	.40	.40	.29			.33
India	.40	1.54	2.95	27.27		2.51
Indonesia		.10	.19			.15
Iran			.04			.03
Iraq			.09			.06
Ireland		.90	.09			.06
Israel	.80		1.26		5.88	1.12
Italy	3.80	7.10	9.78	9.09	5.88	8.54
Japan	10.13	15.55	16.51	4.54		15.64
Korea			.15			.09
Kuwait	.40		.04			.06
Lebanon			.04			.03
Liberia			.04			.03

TABLE V (Continued)

Country	Panel (237)	Proffered Paper (971)	Poster (2065)	Film (22)	Exhibit (17)	Over-all (3312)
Mexico			.09			.06
Netherlands	1.70	.90	.39			.63
New Zealand		.20	.24			.21
Nigeria	.40		.29			.21
Norway	1.26	1.13	1.14			1.12
Paraguay		.10	.09			.09
Peru			.09			.06
Poland			.34			.21
Portugal			.09			.06
Rumania		.40	.82			.63
Saudi Arabia		.20	.34			.27
South Africa	.40	.40	.44	13.64		.42
Spain		.80	.92	4.54		.91
Sweden	1.69	3.30	2.28			2.51
Switzerland	1.26	.80	.53			.69
Tanzania			.04			.03
Thailand	.40					.03
Tunisia		.09				.06
Uganda		.10				.03
United Kingdom	4.64	1.96	1.84			2.05
United States	56.96	45.42	38.06	4.54	82.35	41.61
USSR	.80	.20	.77			.60
Venezuela		.10	.04			.06
Yugoslavia		.30	.92			.69

INDIVIDUALS MEETING THE COMMITMENT
OF A SUBMITTED PAPER

Session	# Scheduled NPC Mtg. 3/82	Cancel- lations	No Shows	Final # Presented	%
Panel 1	7	3		4	
2	8			8	
3	8	1		7	
4	8		2	6	
5	8	1	1	6	
6	8		2	6	
7	8			8	
8	8			8	
9	9			9	
10	8	1		7	
11	8			8	
12	8			8	
13	8	1		7	
14	8			8	
15	8			8	
16	8		1	7	
17	8			8	
18	8	1		7	
19	8			8	
20	8			8	
21	6			6	
22	8			8	
23	8	1		7	
24	8	1		7	
25	8	3		5	
26	8			8	
27	8			8	
28	8	1	1	6	
29	8			8	
30	7			7	
Panel Total	237	14	7	216	91.1

Sessions	# Scheduled NPC Mtg. 3/82	Cancel-lations	No Shows	Final # Presented	%
Proffered					
Paper 1	10			10	
2	10			10	
3	10			10	
4	10			10	
5	10	1		9	
6	10		1	9	
7	10	1	1	8	
8	9		2	7	
9	10		3	7	
10	9	1		8	
11	10	4		6	
12	10	1		9	
13	10			10	
14	10			10	
15	9			9	
16	10		1	9	
17	10			10	
18	10	1		9	
19	10		1	9	
20	9	1		8	
21	10	1		9	
22	7		3	4	
23	10			10	
24	10		1	9	
25	10	1		9	
26	10			10	
27	10	1		9	
28	9	1		8	
29	10			10	
30	10	1	1	9*	
31	8	2		6	
32	10		2	8	
33	10	3	1	6	
34	10			10	
35	10	1	1	8	
36	10			10	
37	10			10	
38	10			10	

Session	# Scheduled NPC Mtg. 3/82	Cancellations	No Shows	Final # Presented	%
Proffered Paper 39	10	1	1	9*	
40	10	2		8	
41	10		4	6	
42	10	1		9	
43	10			10	
44	10		2	8	
45	10			10	
46	10	1		10*	
47	10			10	
48	10	2		9*	
49	10	2	1	8*	
50	10			10	
51	10		1	9	
52	10			10	
53	9			9	
54	10			10	
55	9			9	
56	10			10	
57	10		1	9	
58	10	1	1	8	
59	10			10	
60	10	2		8	
61	10		4	6	
62	9			9	
63	10	1		9	
64	10	1		9	
65	10			10	
66	10			10	
67	10			10	
68	10	1	1	8	
69	10	1	3	6	
70	10		1	9	
71	10			10	
72	10	3		8*	
73	10	1		10*	
74	10			10	
75	10	1	1	8	
76	10			10	

Session	# Scheduled NPC Mtg. 3/82	Cancel- lations	No Shows	Final # Presented	%
Proffered					
Paper 77	10			10	
78	9		2	7	
79	10		1	9	
80	10			10	
81	10			10	
82	10		2	9*	
83	10	2	4	4	
84	10		2	8	
85	9		2	7	
86	10			10	
87	10	1	1	8	
88	9	1		8	
89	10			10	
90	10	1	1	8	
91	10		2	8	
92	10	1		9	
93	10	1	1	8	
94	9			9	
95	10			10	
96	10	3		7	
97	10			10	
98	8	1		7	
99	10			10	
Proffered Paper Total	971	53	57	861	88.7
Panel Total	237	14	7	216	91.1
Grand Total	1208	67	64	1077	89.2

* The discrepancy between the # originally scheduled and the cancel/no show figure is due to the late scheduling of an additional presentation.

BASED ON THE TOTAL NUMBER OF CANCELLATIONS AND NO SHOWS, THE % OF INDIVIDUALS WHO MET THEIR COMMITMENT WAS 89.1 (1077 total presentations + 67 known cancellations and 64 no

shows = 1077/1208 scheduled presentations). THE % WHO DID
NOT MEET THEIR COMMITMENT WAS 19.9.

N.B.: The "no show" figures are based on the Chairman's
Report. Reports on all sessions were not received. It was
not possible to figure the % of poster participants who met
thier commitment since the poster sessions did not have a
Chairperson.

TABLE VII

CANCELLATIONS/REPLACEMENTS AFTER MAY 1, 1982
(INVITED SESSIONS)

Event	Date Cancelled	Replaced by
General Symposium 1*	6/22	P. Shubik
2	7/15	J. Bertino
	6/25	N. Brock
4	8/16	J. Weissberg
5	8/27	W. Myers
6*	8/25	K. Harrap
9	6/27	A. Miller
*	8/15	N. Day
Congress Symposium 2	7/15	G. Cooper
	9/3	J. Bertram
4*	5/14	P. Miescher
*	5/1	S. Ferrone
6	6/25	S. Barranco
8*	8/23	D. Dumonde
12	8/15	M. Iverson
13	5/10	E. Melissinos
19	6/15	D. Park
21*	8/15	T. Phillips
22*	5/1	B. Strauss
26	9/3	H. Takita
28	7/2	C. Land
29	6/25	D. Reede
30	8/20	E. Lotzova
31*	8/25	H. Kaplan
34*	8/13	A. Mantovani
37	5/7	G. Monaco
38	8/17	J. McDougall
43	9/3	T. O'Connor
44	8/20	G. Rovera
Seminar 1	6/30	D. Papahadjopoulos
3*	8/13	P. Burtin
7*	8/5	K. Wiechel
*	7/15	M. Bernardino
	8/15	R. Martin
10	7/22	L. Nadler

TABLE VII (Continued)

Event		Date Cancelled	Replaced by
Seminar	11	8/10	L. Perry
	14	5/9	N. Petrelli
	15	7/15	J. Cassady
		8/15	D. Poplack
	16	6/30	K-H. Robert
		6/5	L. Nadler
	18	7/26	H. Hanafusa
		7/23	L. Rohrscheider
	20	8/18	K. Oho
Round Table	1*	6/3	D. Coffey
	2*	7/14	A. Goldin
	3	5/25	D. Livingston
	8	7/6	C. Maltoni
	14	8/10	C. Smart
	15	8/9	J. Trosko
	18	6/1	M. Rubenstein
	21*	8/25	N. Napalkov
	28	8/18	J. Talmadge
Postgraduate Course	3*	7/6	S. Monfardini
	*	6/25	R. Dorfman
	4*	8/25	D. Haferman
	10*	9/3	B. Pierquin
	12	8/17	N. Samaan
		6/28	A. Spence
	13	8/25	A. Huang
	14	8/25	J. Pickren
		8/13	J. Beckwith
	15	8/25	J. Pickren
	17	9/3	B. Toth
	20	5/22	I. McGregor

Role of Voluntary Societies & Leagues in Cancer Control	2	8/3	P. Hobbs

Plenary Lecture	3	8/25	H. Douglass

TABLE VII (Continued)

Event		Date Cancelled	Replaced by
Proffered Paper			
Session	1*	6/1	K. Munk
	3*	7/4	M. Moore
	14*	7/1	J. Burchenal
	25*	8/31	E. Bjelke
	28*	8/30	W. DeWys
	33*	5/18	K. Munk
	38*	5/10	J. Spratt
	39*	7/29	J. Bowers
	47*	8/16	E. Gillette
	69*	8/10	J. Jessup
	76*	7/15	M. Myers
	85*	8/10	M. Goldrosen
Panel	10*	8/25	M. Mastrangelo
	15*	5/5	H. Wrba
	16*	7/8	H. Koren
	18*	5/1	V. Maher
	22*	6/9	G. Nemeth
	*	8/25	R. Johnson
	27*	6/8	A. Goldstein
	28*	7/6	C. Maltoni

Total: 90/1159 (7.8%)

*Denotes Chariman replacement

The above does not reflect the fact that it was sometimes
necessary to contact several persons in order to find one
that was able to participate.

TABLE VIII

GENERAL REACTION (EVALUATION): COMMENTS EXTRACTED
FROM SESSION CHAIRPERSON REPORTS

GENERAL FAVORABLE COMMENTS

> Well balanced program
> Good discussion
> Presentation of new information
> Good exchange
> Excellent speakers
> Enthusiastic audience
> Filling in time for withdrawn papers done successfully
>   by audience discussion

UNFAVORABLE COMMENTS

> General complaints of lighting (could not be dimmed,
>   only turned out completely)
> Projectionist
> Too much room
> Too little room
> Pointer not working
> Outside noise disturbing (Coliseum rooms)
> Lack of supplies, i.e., chalk, eraser
> Room temperature (too hot or too cold)
> Timer was loud
> Phones not working

SUGGESTIONS: TECHNICAL

> Suggest slide projection be controlled by speaker
> Chairs needed at head table for all speakers to respond
>   to questions from stage
> Light switch should be next to projector or at front
>   of room

TABLE VIII (Continued)

SUGGESTIONS: PROGRAM

　　　Suggest similar symposium at next Congress (GS-3:
　　　　Advances in Diagnosis and Staging)
　　　No time allowed for discussion in Postgraduate Course 6
　　　　(discussion was wanted by audience)
　　　Poor attendance (P-21:   Interferon)
　　　Abstracts poorly presented (P-21:   Interferon)
　　　Language problems (P-21:   Interferon)
　　　Disappointing quality of several papers (PPS-53: BRM II)

89.8% (115/128 panel and proffered paper sessions) were
returned to the office of the Program Chairman

EVALUATION OF PROGRAM BALANCE

	Carcino-genesis	Epidemiology	Treatment Preclin.	Clin.	Biology of Disease & Basic Res.	Immunology Preclin. & Clinical	Diagnostics	Allied Sciences	Total Number
General Symposia	1	0	1	2	1	1	2	1	9
Symposia	4	1	2	13	18	5	2	3	48
Postgraduate Courses	0	0	0	16	1	0	1	2	20
Seminars	0	0	1	7	3	5	1	4	21
Round Tables	6	3	3	6	8	1	1	3	31
Panels	1	1	0	9	8	7	2	2	30
Proffered Paper Session	7	5	11	41	15	9	6	5	99
Posters	8	5	9	23	13	18	7	6	89
Role of Volunteer Society	0	0	0	0	0	0	0	10	10
Films	0	0	0	8	0	0	1	0	9
Special Sessions	0	0	0	2	0	0	0	0	2
Plenary Lectures	1	1	0	5	1	1	0	2	11
TOTALS:	28	16	27	132	68	47	23	38	379

C. Countries Represented at the 13th International Cancer Congress

Eighty-four (84) countries were represented at the 13th International Cancer Congress in Seattle, Washington, USA:

3-Algeria	1-Ivory Coast	1-Tonga
98-Argentina	2-Jamaica	1-Trinidad
103-Australia	929-Japan	4-Tunisia
42-Austria	1-Kenya	2703-United
1-Bahrain	9-Korea	States
22-Belgium	7-Kuwait	7-USSR
8-Bolivia	12-Lebanon	1-Uganda
78-Brazil	1-Liberia	5-Uruguay
2-Bulgaria	1-Libya	20-Venezuela
201-Canada	4-Malaysia	2-West Indies
10-Chile	21-Mexico	40-Yugoslavia
10-Colombia	96-Netherlands	1-Zimbabwe
1-Costa Rica	23-New Zealand	
7-Cuba	11-Nigeria	
5-Czechoslovakia	74-Norway	
54-Denmark	1-Pakistan	
2-Dominican	10-Panama	
Republic	6-Paraguay	
31-Egypt	22-Peoples' Republic	
137-England	of China	
2-Ecuador	11-Peru	
207-Federal Republic	3-Philippines	
of Germany	7-Poland	
33-Finland	23-Portugal	
170-France	10-Puerto Rico	
11-German Democratic	1-Qatar	
Republic	45-Republic of	
24-Greece	South Africa	
1-Guam	1-Rumania	
3-Hong Kong	11-Saudi Arabia	
13-Hungary	12-Scotland	
14-Iceland	3-Singapore	
57-India	38-Spain	
36-Indonesia	3-Suriname	
9-Iran	158-Sweden	
6-Iraq	57-Switzerland	
8-Ireland	19-Taiwan	
48-Israel	1-Tanzania	
262-Italy	12-Thailand	

D. Press Room Report

SUMMARY:

One hundred and fifty (150) media members attended the
Congress. Coverage by newspapers, magazines, medical
journals, television and radio was extensive. The
United States, Great Britain, Japan, Luxembourg, Brazil
and Sweden provided television coverage; eight features
on cancer developments were filmed by a local television
company; NBC filmed five 30-minute programs. The
Congress Press Room facilities were deemed excellent by
the press members.

Press Room Report

The Congress Press Room was a successful operation; the
stories generated there contributed to dissemination of
current developments in cancer treatment and control to
a world-wide lay and professional audience.

One hundred and fifty (150) writers, photographers and
television reporters made full use of the press room.
Many expressed their pleasure with the facilities and
services provided.

A computer readout listing delegates and their Congress
addresses enabled press room and message center staff to
reach most of those individuals requested for interview
by members of the press.

The press room staff comprised of two public relations
professionals, two assistants, a receptionist, copy
machine operator and telex/telecopier operator and two
volunteers. Press room hours were from 7:30 am to 8:00
or 9:00 pm, starting September 7th through 15th. The
National Cancer Institute and the American Cancer society
each supplied a volunteer who helped locate and schedule
interviews for briefings by scientific members from their
respective organizations.

The Congress issue of the Cancer Letter was produced from
the Congress Press Room, as were the on-site issues of
the Congress newspaper, produced by Academy Professional
Information Services.

          Prepared by: Georgia Gellert and Joan McKay

E.   Special Meetings and Functions

A number of meetings, seminars and educational programs
were conducted at local hotels during the course of the
Congress by various organizations:

International Union Against Cancer

- Council Nominating Committee
- Membership Committee
- Finance Committee
- Outgoing Council
- Honors and Awards Committee
- UICC Foundation
- General Assembly
- USA Committee to UICC
- Professional Education Committee
- Incoming Council
- Incoming Executive Committee

International Association of Cancer Registries
Veterans Administration Oncology Group
International Society of Radiation Oncologists
Association of American Cancer Institutes/UICC Committee
   on International Collaborative Activities (AACI/CICA)
Oiland Shriner Lectures - Fred Hutchinson Cancer
   Research Center
American Association of Cancer Education
Oncology Nursing - Education Committee
Centralized Cancer Patient Data System
Mead Johnson Pharmaceutical Division
NIH Toxicology Data Bank Review Committee
Oncology Editorial Board
M.D. Anderson Hospital and Tumor Institute Alumni
International Council-Society of Pathology
The Prostate Editorial Board
American Joint Committee on Cancer
The President's Cancer Panel
International Journal of Cancer
Damon Runyon-Walter Winchell Fund Board
General Motors Awards Assembly
Lederle Laboratories
Parke-Davis Co.
Ciba Pharmaceutical Co.

F. Exhibits

SUMMARY

One hundred and ten (110) commerical exhibits occupied
160 10' x 8' booths in the 40,000 square foot Exhibition
Hall at the Seattle Center. The Exhibition Hall also
housed the message center and post office and banking
facilities for the convenience of delegates. The
commercial exhibition was managed by Steven K. Herlitz,
Inc., New York.

The Secretary-General's impression was that, despite
the difficult economic climate, exhibit sales were
excellent.

Sixteen organizations exhibited scientific displays in
individual booths located in the Coliseum, adjacent to
the scientific poster sessions.

COMMERCIAL EXHIBITORS

ADAC LABORATORIES
ABBOTT LABORATORIES
ACADEMIC BOOK EXHIBITS
ADRIA LABORATORIES
ALPHA OMEGA SERVICES, INC.
ALZA CORPORATION
AMERICAN PHARMASEAL (KORMED)
ARMOUR PHARMACEUTICAL CO.
AUTO-SYRINGE, INC.
AVANTI POLAR LIPIDS
BIO-SCIENCES INFORMATION SERVICE
BSL TECHNOLOGY
BSD MEDICAL CORPORATION
BAKER INSTRUMENT CORPORATION
BAUSCH & LOMB
BECTION DICKINSON FACS SYSTEMS
BEECHAM LABORATORIES
BEST INDUSTRIES
BIOMOLECULAR DYNAMICS
BIOMED MEDICAL MANUFACTURING COMPANY
BRISTOL LABORATORIES
BURROUGHS, WELLCOME COMPANY
CGR MED
CALBIOCHEM-BEHRING CORPORATION

CASCADE X-RAY SPECIALISTS
CGL-CONSOLIDATED BIOMEDICAL LABORATORIES
CHURCHILL LIVINGSTON, INC.
CIBA-GEIGY
CLAY-ADAMS (BECTON DICKINSON)
COHERENT, INC.
COLD SPRING HARBOR LABORATORIES
CORMED, INC.
COULTER ELECTRONICS
DAKO CORPORATION
DUPONT COMPANY (Sorvall Division)
DYNATECH LABORATORIES
ELI LILLY & COMPANY
ELM SERVICES, INC.
ENCYCLOPEDIA BRITTANICA, USA
EVERGREEN MEDICAL PRODUCTS
E-Y LABORATORIES
FENWAL LABORATORIES (Travenol)
CAMMEX, INC.
GENETIC SYSTEMS CORPORATION
GERMFREE LABORATORIES
GRUNE & STRATTON, INC.
HAEMONETICS CORPORATION
HALL, G.K. & COMPANY
HEINICKLE INSTRUMENTS CO. (National Appliance)
HELENA LABORATORIES
HEMED, INC.
HOECHST-ROUSSEL PHARMACEUTICALS
HOEFFER SCIENTIFIC INSTRUMENTS
HOSPITAL CORPORATION INTERNATIONAL
INFUSAID CORPORATION
INTERNATIONAL INSTRUMENTS FOR MEDICAL SCIENCE
IVES LABORATORIES
JANSSEN PHARMACEUTICA
JORDON SCIENTIFIC
KARGER PUBLISHERS, INC.
KAY LABORATORIES
KNOLL PHARMACEUTICALS COMPANY
LEA AND FEBIGER
LEDERLE LABORATORIES
LEITZ, F. INC.
LIPPINCOTT, J.B. & COMPANY
LISS, ALAN R. INC.
LUNING PARK ASSOCIATES, INC.
MARTINUS NIJHOFF MEDICAL PUBLISHER
MASSON PUBLISHING USA, INC.

McGRAW-HILL BOOK COMPANY
MEAD JOHNSON PHARAMCEUTICALS
MEDICAL ASSOCIATES INTERNATIONAL
MILES PHARMACEUTICALS
MOSBY LABORATORIES
NBBJ GROUP
NEUTRON PRODUCTS, INC.
NEW ENGLAND NUCLEAR CORPORATION
NIKON, INC.
NORFOLK MEDICAL PRODUCTS, INC.
NU AIRE, INC.
NU TECH MEDICAL SYSTEMS, INC.
NUCLETRONIX, INC.
ONCOLOGY LABORATORIES, INC.
ONCOLOGY NURSING SOCIETY
OMIMETRIX
ORGANON, INC.
PARKE DAVIS (Warner Lambert)
PERGAMON PRESS, INC.
PHARMACIA, INC.
POLARON INSTRUMENTS
QUEST MEDICAL, INC.
QUESTEL, INC.
RAVEN PRESS
RIBI IMMUNO CHEM RESEARCH, INC.
ROBBINS, A.H., INC.
ROSS LABORATORIES (Division of Abbott)
SAUNDERS, W.B. CO.
SCIENTIFIC RESOURCE ASSOCIATES
SIEMANS CORPORATION
SOREDEX/UNITAS
SPRINGER-BERLAG NEW YROK, INC.
STUART PHARMACEUTICALS
TAGO, INC.
VARIAN ASSOCIATION
VECTOR LABORATORIES
UHI CORPORATION
WESCOR, INC.
ZYMED LABORATORIES
CENTOCAR, INC.

SCIENTIFIC EXHIBITORS

AMERICAN CANCER SOCIETY
AMERICAN ASSOCIATION FOR CANCER EDUCATION
ASSOCIATION OF COMMUNITY CANCER CENTERS

GUTTMAN INSTITUTE AND THE GEORGETOWN UNIVERSITY AND
   UCLA SCHOOLS OF MEDICINE
COMMISSION ON CANCER OF THE COLLEGE OF SURGEONS,
   AMERICAN JOINT COMMITTEE ON CANCER
FRED HUTCHINSON CANCER RESEARCH CENTER
INTERNATIONAL UNION AGAINST CANCER (UICC)
NEW YORK METROPOLITAN BREAST CANCER GROUP, INC.
NATIONAL CANCER INSTITUTE
NATIONAL LARGE BOWEL CANCER PROJECT, THE UNIVERSITY OF
   TEXAS SYSTEM CANCER CENTER, M.D. ANDERSON HOSPITAL
   AND TUMOR INSTITUTE
NATIONAL PROSTATIC CANCER PROJECT
NEW YORK STATE CANCER PROGRAMS ASSOCIATION, INC.
PACIFIC NORTHWEST RESEARCH COMMISSION
THE SWEDISH HOSPITAL TUMOR INSTITUTE
VETERANS ADMINISTRATION HOSPITAL (NY)
VIRGINIA MASON MEDICAL CENTER

G. Office of the Secretariat

Secretary-General - Dr. Edwin A. Mirand

<u>Seattle Office</u>

1.   Karen Craig
2.   Sara Gertsner
3.   Douglas Marshall
4.   Anne Marie Murphy
5.   Bridget Murphy
6.   Margaret Murphy
7.   Jan Peischel
8.   David Siegel
9.   Jeffrey Spellman
10. Teresa Spellman
11. Margo Spellman-Tagas
12. Anne Tee

<u>Buffalo Office</u>

13. Lisa Barone
14. Linda Beverage
15. Kevin Craig
16. Lois Earsing
17. Judy Felski
18. Marge Foti
19. Ann Gannon
20. Bonnie Glenn
21. Robert Hall
22. Teena Holder
23. Craig Johnson
24. Nina Johnston
25. Colleen Karuza
26. Linda McKernan
27. Ramon Melendez
28. Catherine O'Leary
29. James Peterson
30. Carole Pieroni
31. Maureen Schubauer
32. Deborah Study
33. Dan Terrana
34. Helen Vlahopoulos
35. Irene Wieczorek
36. Elena Musmanno

H. Committees of the Congress

The structure of the 13th International Cancer Congress
included a National Organizing Committee, National
Program Committee, International Scientific Advisory
Board and the Pacific Northwest Local Organizing
Committee. Congress officers included Dr. William B.
Hutchinson, President; Hon. Warren G. Magnuson, Honorary
President; Dr. Edwin A. Mirand, Secretary-General;
Mr. Lane Adams, Honorary Vice President; Dr. R. Lee
Clark, Honorary Vice President and Dr. Arthur C. Upton,
Honorary Vice President.

The purpose of the National Organizing Committee was to
establish the broad policies of the Congress. The
National Program Committee and the International
Scientific Advisory Board established the scientific
program. The Pacific Northwest Local Organizing
Committee recommended the social program and advised
on local arrangements.

NATIONAL ORGANIZING COMMITTEE

Dr. William B. Hutchinson
Chairman
Fred Hutchinson Cancer
  Research Center
1124 Columbia Street
Seattle, WA 98104
(Ph: 206, 292-2930

Dr. Edwin A. Mirand
Co-Chairman
Roswell Park Memorial Inst.
666 Elm Street
Buffalo, NY 14263
(Ph: 716, 845-3028)

Dr. Richard F. Bakemeier
Associate Director
University of Rochester
  Cancer Center
601 Elmwood Avenue
Box 704
Rochester, NY 14642
(Ph: 716, 275-5537)

Mrs. Helene G. Brown
Executive Director
Community Cancer Control/
  Los Angeles, Inc.
5800 Wilshire Boulevard
Los Angeles, CA 90036
(Ph: 213, 938-2608

Dr. Stephen K. Carter
Director
Northern California Cancer
  Program
P.O. Box 10144
Palo Alto, CA 94303
(Ph: 415, 497-7431

Dr. Robert C. Coe
1117 Columbia Street
Seattle, WA 98104

Dr. Murray M. Copeland
Vice-President
University Cancer Foundation
The Univ. of Texas System
  Cancer Center
M.D. Anderson Hospital and
  Tumor Institute
Texas Medical Center
Houston, TX 77030
(Ph: 713, 792-3025)

Dr. Hugh J. Creech
American Association for
  Cancer Research
Fox Chase Cancer Center
7701 Burholme Avenue
Philadelphia, PA 19111
(Ph: 215, 728-2455)

Dr. Gale Katterhagen
Director of Oncology
Tacoma General Hospital
315 South K. Street
Tacoma, WA 98405
(Ph: 206, 597-7700)

Dr. LaSalle D. Leffall, Jr.
Professor and Chairman
Department of Surgery
Howard University
College of Medicine
Washington, DC 20059
(Ph: 202, 745-1441)

Dr. Enrico Mihich
Roswell Park Memorial Inst.
666 Elm Street
Buffalo, NY 14263
(Ph: 716, 845-5759)

Dr. Daniel G. Miller
Director
Preventive Medicine Inst.
Strang Clinic
55 East 34th Street
New York, NY 10016
(212, 683-1000)

Dr. Robert W. Miller
Chief, Clinical Epidemi-
  ology Branch
Acting Associate Director
  for International
  Affairs
National Cancer Institute
Rm. A521, Landow Bldg.
Bethesda, MD 20205
(Ph: 301, 496-5785)

Dr. W.P. Laird Myers
Memorial Sloan-Kettering
  Institute
1275 York Avenue
New York, NY 10021
(Ph: 212, 794-8380)

Dr. Gregory T. O'Conor
Director
Division of Cancer Cause
  and Prevention
National Cancer Institute
Bldg. 31, Rm. 11A19
Bethesda, MD 20205
(Ph: 301, 496-6618)

Dr. Albert H. Owens, Jr.
Director
John's Hopkins Oncology
  Center
600 North Wolfe Street
Baltimore, MD 21205
(Ph: 301, 955-8822)

Dr. Henry C. Pitot
Director
McArdle Laboratory for
  Cancer Research
Medical Center
University of Wisconsin
Madison, WI 53706
(Ph: 608,262-2177)

Dr. William W. Shingleton
Director
Duke Comprehensive Cancer Ctr.
Duke University Medical Ctr.
P.O. Box 3814
Durham, NC 27710
(Ph: 919, 684-2282)

Dr. Willis Taylor
Virginia Mason Clinic
1118 Ninth Avenue
Seattle, WA 98101

Dr. George Weber
Professor and Director
Laboratory for Experimental
  Oncology
Indiana University School
  of Medicine
1100 West Michigan Street
Indianapolis, IN 46223
(Ph: 317, 264-7921)

Mr. Francis J. Wilcox
Wilcox and Wilcox
Suite 500-504
131 South Barstow Street
Eau Claire, WI 54701
(Ph: 715, 832-6645)

NATIONAL PROGRAM COMMITTEE

Dr. Enrico Mihich
Chairman
Director of Experimental
  Therapeutics and Grace
  Cancer Drug Center
Roswell Park Memorial Inst.
666 Elm Street
Buffalo, NY 14263
(Ph: 716, 845-5759)

Dr. William W. Shingleton
Vice-Chairman
Director, Duke Comprehensive
  Cancer Center
Durham, NC 27710
(Ph: 919, 684-3895)

Dr. Renato Baserga
Temple University School
  of Medicine
Philadelphia, PA 19140
(Ph: 215, 221-3257)

Dr. Paul P. Carbone
Wisconsin Clinical Cancer
  Center
University of Wisconsin
Department of Human Onc.
600 Highland Avenue
Madison, WI 53792
(Ph: 608, 263-8600)

Dr. Edward Copeland, III
University of Texas
M.D. Anderson Hospital &
  Tumor Institute
Texas Medical Center
Houston, TX 77025
(Ph: 713, 792-5405)

Dr. Gerald Dodd
University of Texas
M.D. Anderson Hospital &
  Tumor Institute
Texas Medical Center
Houston, TX 77025
(Ph: 713, 792-2700)

Dr. Diane Fink
Div. of Cancer Control &
  Rehabilitation
National Cancer Institute
Bethesda, MD 20014
(Ph: 301, 427-7997)

Dr. Joseph F. Fraumeni, Jr.
National Institutes of Health
U.S. Public Health Service
Landow Building
Bethesda, MD 20205
(Ph: 301, 496-1691)

Dr. Harry V. Gelboin, Chief
Chemistry Branch
National Cancer Institute
Bethesda, MD 20205
(Ph: 301, 496-6716, 6849)

Dr. Karl Hellstrom
Fred Hutchinson Cancer
  Research Center
1124 Columbia Street
Seattle, WA 98104
(Ph: 206, 292-2667)

Dr. Evan Hersh
University of Texas
M.D. Anderson Hospital &
  Tumor Institute
Texas Medical Center
Houston, TX 77025
(Ph: 713, 792-3200)

Dr. Robert C. Hickey
University of Texas
M.D. Anderson Hospital &
    Tumor Institute
Texas Medical Center
Houston, TX 77025
(Ph: 713, 792-3200)

Dr. Arthur I. Holleb
American Cancer Society, Inc
777 Third Avenue
New York, NY 10017
(Ph: 212, 867-3700)

Dr. Frank M. Huennekens
Dept. of Biochemistry
Scripps Clinic and
  Research Foundation
LaJolla, CA 92037
(Ph: 714, 454-3881)

Dr. Robert V.P. Hutter
Dept. of Pathology
St. Barnabas Medical Center
Old Short Hills Road
Livingston, NJ 07039
(Ph: 201, 533-5750)

Dr. Simon Kramer
Dept. of Radiation Therapy
  & Nuclear Medicine
Jefferson Medical College
Thomas Jefferson Univ.
Philadelphia, PA 19107
(Ph: 215, 928-6700)

Dr. John Laszlo
Duke Medical Center
Duke University
Durham, NC 27710
(Ph: 919, 684-6450)

Dr. Ronald Malt
Massachusetts General Hospital
Boston, MA 02114
(Ph: 617, 726-2821)

INTERNATIONAL SCIENTIFIC ADVISORY BOARD

Dr. William B. Hutchinson
  Chairman, USA

Dr. Edwin A. Mirand
  Co-Chairman, USA

Dr. Umberto Veronesi
  Ex-Officio, Italy

Dr. Gerald P. Murphy
  Ex-Officio, USA

Dr. Salomon Barg
  Argentina

Dr. Jean Bernard
  France

Dr. Eduardo Caceres
  Peru

Dr. R. Lee Clark
  USA

Dr. G. Della Porta
  Italy

Dr. Jerzy Einhorn
  Sweden

Dr. Ismail El-Sebai
  Egypt

Dr. Peter H. Fitzgerald
  New Zealand

Dr. Silvio Garattini
  Italy

Dr. Frans Geldenmuys
  South Africa

Dr. Kenneth Harrap
  England

Dr. Hung-Chiu Ho
  Hong Kong

Dr. Dareb Jussawalla
  India

Dr. R. A. MacBeth
  Canada

Dr. Enrico Mihich
  USA

Dr. Julio Ospina
  Colombia

Dr. A. Pihl
  Norway

Dr. Gordon Sarfaty
  Australia

Dr. Carl Schmidt
  Federal Republic of Germany

Dr. Ciro Servadio
  Israel

Dr. Wu Huan Sing
  China

Dr. Takashi Sugimura
  Japan

Dr. Henri J. Tagnon
  Belgium

Sr. S. Tanneberger
  Dem. Republic of Germany

Dr. N. Trapeznikov
  USSR

Dr. M. Tubiana
  France

Dr. A. Olufemi Williams
  Nigeria

Dr. Henrich Wrba
  Austria

OFFICERS

Dr. William B. Hutchinson, President

Hon. Warren G. Magnuson, Honorary President

Dr. Edwin A. Mirand, Secretary-General

Mr. Lane Adams, Honorary Vice-President

Dr. R. Lee Clark, Honorary Vice-President

Dr. Arthur C. Upton, Honorary Vice-President

BOARD OF TRUSTEES

Dr. William B. Hutchinson

Dr. Edwin A. Mirand

Dr. Stephen K. Carter

Mr. David C. Lycette

Mr. Francis J. Wilcox

Index

Adjuvant and multimodal treatment
    trials, 33–39
American Cancer Society, 9–10, 150–
    151
    and cancer epidemiology, 83
    Reach for Recovery, 27
Antivivisectionists, 96
Arabinosyl cytosine, 57, 58
Argentina, 7
Asbestos, 72, 78, 92

Betel nut, 72
Blood aplasia, 125–126
Bone marrow grafting/transplant, 125–
    126
    graft material, 133
    and intensive chemotherapy in
        disseminated malignant
        disease, 133–137
Brazil, 7
Breast
    cancer, 49
        lymph node involvement and
            recurrence, 51
        radiation oncology, 115–116
        mastectomy, 31–32
        self-examination, public education,
            26–27

Cable Health Network and Cable News
    Network, 159
Canada, 12, 18
Cancer
    care coordination
        centralized data registry, 11
        elements of comprehensive
            programs, 16, 21
        forerunners of modern
            approaches, 4

fund raising, 19
inter-institutional research
    integration, 4–5
International Directory, 21
international exchange, 5–6, 13–
    18
national collaborative treatment
    groups, 16, 21
national efforts, 6–10
national standards of care, 10–11
national stimulation of local
    initiatives, 13
nineteenth century cf. modern
    organization, 3–4
regional associations, 7
specialized services and referral
    networks, 12, 17
center, comprehensive, UICC
    guidelines, 20
congresses, 26
control
    non-medical organization, role of,
        27–29
    organization, role of, 25–29
epidemiology. *See* Epidemiology,
    epidemiology
journals, 4, 7
    in which Congress was
        highlighted, 160–161
prevention, 28
registration, 74–75
surgeon. *See* Surgical oncology
see also specific cancer sites and
    types
Carcinogenesis
    and epidemiology, 71–72
    schema, 71
    see also Epidemiology, cancer;
        Tumor promotion

Carcinogens, 81
Carcinoma, primary hepatocellular, 73
Cesium seeds, 110–111; *see also*
   Radiation oncology
Chemoprevention, 86
Chemotherapy
   adjuvant, 54
   combined modality treatment, 49,
      54–62
   failure, 47
   Goldie-Coldman model, 57, 58, 62–
      64
   intensive, and bone marrow
      transplant in disseminated
      malignant disease, 133–137
   long-term infusion, 40–42
   metastases, 48
      multiple, 59–60
   phases in development, 50
   resistance, 47, 56
      causes, 52
      spontaneous development of
         phenotypic resistance, 62–
         64
      and tumor mass, 56–62
   and tumor
      doubling times, 53–55
      mass-prognosis relationship, 47,
         49–50, 53, 55–56
   see also Radiation oncology, Surgical
      oncology
Chile, 7
China, 9
Chromates, 72
Chromosome, Philadelphia, 135
Cigarettes. *See* Smoking
Cobalt radiotherapy, 48
Coffee, 91, 100
Colombia, 8, 12, 14–15
Combined modality treatment, 49,
   54–62; *see also* Chemotherapy
Communicable diseases, 9
Congresses, cancer, 4, 26; *see also*
   Thirteenth International
      Cancer Congress
Coordination. *See* Cancer care
   coordination

Costa Rica, 8
CT scan, 110; *see also* Radiation
   oncology
Cyclophosphamide, 57, 60, 135
Cyclosporine, 135, 136
Cytomegalovirus, 136

Data registry, centralized, 11; *see also*
   Cancer care coordination
Debulking, 60
Developing world
   communicable diseases, 9
   smoking in, 94–95
   see also specific countries
Diet, 79–81
Disease(s)
   communicable, 9
   graft vs. host, 126, 134–137
Drug resistance phenotype
   genetic origin, 63
   spontaneous development, 62–64

Education, public
   breast self-examination, 26–27
   cancer epidemiology, 95–96
Epidemiology, cancer
   ACS, 83
   barriers to progress, 86–93
      access to tools of trade, 89–90
      computers and statistics, 93
      identification of migrants, 88–89
      observational cf. experimental,
         86–87
      parochialism, 87–88, 100
      small relative risk, 91–92
   carcinogens, 81
   chemoprevention, 86
   Clearing House, 82
   current, 74–77
      cancer registration, 74–75
      descriptive vs. analytic, 74, 77
      maps, 75–76
      relative frequency, 76
      standardization, 76–77
      time trends, 76
   diet, 79–81
   future prospects, 83–86

genetic susceptibility, 99–100
informing the public, 96–98
international studies needed, 87–88
lifestyle factors, 72–73, 79–80, 99
occupation, 77–78
past history, 72–74, 98
place in carcinogenesis, 71–72
priorties, 73–83, 99
research funding, 82–83
risk
  /benefit analysis, 97–98
  factors, 73
  relative, small, 91–92
susceptibility, 85
tumor promotion, 84–85
UICC Committee on Geographical
  Pathology, 74

Final report. *See* Thirteenth
  International Cancer Congress
  Final Report
Fluoride in drinking water, 96
Food and Agriculture Organization
  (FAO), 94
Fractionation, 108–109; *see also*
  Radiation oncology
Funding/fund raising
  cancer care coordination, 19
  cancer epidemiology, 82–83

Gastric cancer and resection
  curative, definition, 33–35
  Japan cf. U.S., 35–37, 44
Genetic
  origin of drug-resistant phenotype,
    63
  susceptibility, 99–100
P-Glycoprotein, 63
Gompertzian growth kinetics, 51
Grafting, bone marrow. *See* Bone
  marrow grafting/transplant
Graft vs. host disease, 126, 134–137

Heidelberger, Charles, 163
Hepatocellular carcinoma, primary, 73
Hyperbaric oxygen, 120; *see also*
  Radiation oncology

Hyperthermia, 117–118
Hypoxia, 120–122

Iceland, 86
Industrialization, 9
Interferon, 136
International Agency for Cancer
  Research, 6
International Cancer Research Data
  Bank, 6
International Classification of Diseases,
  77
International exchange, 13–18; *see also*
  Cancer care coordination
International oncology, cancer care
  coordination, 5–6
International Union Against Cancer
  (UICC), 5, 9, 17, 148–149
  Committee on Geographical
    Pathology, 74
  guidelines for developing a
    comprehensive cancer center,
    20
  1981 Advisory Meeting, 21–22
  traditional pattern of organization,
    25–26
  see also Thirteenth International
    Cancer Congress Final Report
Iridium wires, 110–111

Japan, gastric cancer and resection, cf.
  U.S., 35–37, 44
Jaundice, 43–44
Journals, cancer, 4, 7
  in which Congress was highlighted,
    160–161

Kinetics, tumor cell, 51, 122–123

Latin America. *See* specific countries
Leukemia
  acute, 133–134, 137
  chronic myelogenous, 135–136
Lifestyle factors, 72–73, 79–80, 99
Liver
  metastases, 39–42
  primary hepatocellular carcinoma, 73

Local initiatives, national stimulation, 13; *see also* Cancer care coordination
Lung metastases, 41, 43, 115
Lymphomas, 60, 61

Manpower and epidemiology, 90–91
Maps, cancer epidemiological, 75–76
Mastectomy, 31–32
Media coverage of Congress 158–159
Metastases
  and chemotherapy, 48
  liver, 39–42
  micro-, labelling indices, 54, 115
  multiple, and chemotherapy, 59–60
  pulmonary, 41, 43, 115
Metastic disease and surgical oncology, 39–44
Methotrexate, 135, 136
Mexico, 8
Micrometastases, labelling indices, 54
Migrants, identification of, in epidemiology, 88–89
Multimodal and adjuvant treatment trials, 33–39
Mutation rate, 61

β-Naphthylamines, 72
National Cancer Act (U.S., 1971), 9
National Cancer Institute, 6, 18
  SEER, 49
National collaborative treatment groups, 18–19; *see also* Cancer care coordination
National efforts, standards. *See* Cancer care coordination
National Public Radio, 159
Nitrosamines, 80

Occupation, 77–78
Oncogenes, 47, 64–65
Oncology. *See* Radiation oncology, Surgical oncology
Organization of Economic Cooperation and Development (OECD), 82
Organization, role in cancer control, 25–29

non-medical, 27–29
Osteosarcoma, 37–39
Oxygen, hyperbaric, 120; *see also* Radiation oncology

Pain killing by radiation, 125
Parochialism and cancer epidemiology, 87–88, 100
Particle therapy, 120–122; *see also* Radiation oncology
Passive smoking, 91, 100; *see also* Smoking
Pathologic fractures, 43
Peru, 8, 17–18
Petronius, 83
Phenotypic resistance. *See* Chemotherapy
Philadelphia chromosome, 135
Plenary lectures, summary, 154–155
Press coverage of Congress, 158–159
Press room, Congress, 158
  report, 193
Prevention, cancer, 28
Professional societies, 4
Prognosis–tumor mass relationship, 47, 49–50, 53, 55–56
Proton beam, 111; *see also* Radiation oncology
Publications, 155; *see also* Journals, cancer
Pulmonary metastases, 41, 43, 115

Radiation exposure, 92
Radiation oncology, 107–127
  blood aplasia risk, 125–126
  breast cancer, 115–116
  bulky tumors, 114
  cesium seeds, 110–111
  with chemotherapy, 107, 116–117
  clinical dosimetry, 109
  cobalt, 48
  complication rates, factors affecting, 112
  CT scan, 110
  different patterns of spread, 123–124
  fractionation, 108–119
  future, 118–119

history, 107–118
  mature phase (1955–1980), 109–118
  modern, birth of, 108–109
hyperbaric oxygen, 120
hyperthermia, 117–118
hypoxia, 120–122
individualization of treatment, 124–125
institutional variability, 113
intraoperative, 111
intrinsic radioresistance, 123
iridium wires, 110–111
megavoltage, 109–111
pain killing, 125
particle therapy, 120–122
prognostic factors, 124–125
prophylaxis for pulmonary
  micrometastases, 115
proton beam, 111
quality control, 111–113
radiobiology impact, 113–116
radioresistance of human tumors,
  119–120
shrinking field technique, 115
with surgery, 107
total body irradiation in generalized
  disease, 125–126
tumor cell kinetics, 122–123
tumor localization, 110
see also Chemotherapy, Surgical
  oncology
Radiobiology, 113–116
Reach for Recovery, 27
Recurrent disease and surgical oncology,
  39–44
Referral networks, 12, 17; see also
  Cancer care coordination
Regional association, 7
Registration, cancer, 74–75
Risk
  /benefit analysis and cancer
    epidemiology, 97–98
  factors, 73

Sanctuaries, tumor cell, 47–49, 52–53
Scandinavia, 15, 16

Self-examination, breast, 26–27
Singapore, 9
Smoking, 17, 72, 99
  in developing world, 94–95
  passive, 91, 100
  and UN and FAO, 94
Subspecialty groups, 31
Surgical oncology, 31–44
  adjuvant and multimodal treatment
    trials, 33–39
  cf. cancer surgeon, 32–33
  future, 44
  gastric cancer, 33–37
  osteosarcoma, 37–39
  recurrent and metastic disease, 39–44
  see also Chemotherapy, Radiation
    oncology
Swedish Cancer Society, 19

Thirteenth International Cancer
  Congress Final Report, 145–165,
  192–207
  accomodations, 157
  ACS, 150–151
  attendance, 155–156
  background, 148–150
  closing ceremony, 164
  committees of the Congress, 200
  communications, 157–158
  countries represented, 192
  exhibits, 195–198
    commercial, 195–197
    scientific, 197–198
  funding sources, 165
  International Scientific Advisory
    Board, listed, 205–206
  journals in which Congress was
    highlighted, 160–161
  local organizing committee, 161
  media coverage, 158–159
  Mucio Athyade Prize, 163
  National Organizing Committee, 149
    listed, 201–202
  National Program Committee, 150
    listed, 203–204
  see also Thirteenth International

Cancer Congress National
Program Committee Report
officers, listed, 207
opening ceremony, 163–164
organizations, listed, 194
participating nonphysicians, 150
press room, 158
report, 193
promotional efforts, 159–161
publications, 155
scientific program, 150–155, 166–
191
disease management, 151–154
plenary lectures, 154–155
see also Thirteenth International
Cancer Congress National
Program Committee Report
Secretariat (Buffalo and Seattle), 199
security, 158
site, 156
social program, 161–162
special meetings and functions, 194
staffing, 164–165
transportation, 157
travel coordinator, 156–157
UICC, 148–149
volunteer participation, 161–163
Thirteenth International Cancer
Congress National Program
Committee Report, 166–191
abstract rejections, 174
cancellations/replacements after
May 1, 1982, 186–188
changes made during Congress, 171
general reaction evaluation, 189–190
individuals meeting commitment of
submitted paper, 181–185
invited sections, 172–173
program balance, 189, 191
submitted sections, 175–176
as percent of event total, 179–180
total presentations of countries by

event, 177–178
summary, 167, 169–171
see also Thirteenth International
Cancer Congress Final Report
Tobacco. See Smoking
α-Tocopherol, 86
Transplants, bone marrow. See Bone
marrow grafting/transplant
Trials, adjuvant and multimodal
treatment, and
surgical oncology, 33–39
Tumor(s)
cell
kinetics, 122–123
sanctuaries, 47–49, 52–53
doubling times, 53–55
mass–prognosis relationship, 47, 49–
50, 53, 55–56;
see also Chemotherapy
promoter identification, 85
promotion, 84–85

UICC. See International Union Against
Cancer
United Kingdom, 88–89
United Nations, 94
United States, 8, 9
bilateral agreements with other
national cancer agencies, 14
gastric cancer and resection, cf.
Japan, 35–37, 44
see also specific agencies
Uruguay, 8

Venezuela, 8
Vinyl chloride, 91
Virus, CMV, 136
Vitamins A and C, 86
Voluntary agencies, 4

Water, drinking, fluoride in, 96
World Health Organization, 6, 10

PROGRESS IN CLINICAL AND BIOLOGICAL RESEARCH

Series Editors

Nathan Back
George J. Brewer
Vincent P. Eijsvoogel
Robert Grover

Kurt Hirschhorn
Seymour S. Kety
Sidney Udenfriend
Jonathan W. Uhr

Vol 1: **Erythrocyte Structure and Function,** George J. Brewer, *Editor*

Vol 2: **Preventability of Perinatal Injury,** Karlis Adamsons, Howard A. Fox, *Editors*

Vol 3: **Infections of the Fetus and the Newborn Infant,** Saul Krugman, Anne A. Gershon, *Editors*

Vol 4: **Conflicts in Childhood Cancer: An Evaluation of Current Management,** Lucius F. Sinks, John O. Godden, *Editors*

Vol 5: **Trace Components of Plasma: Isolation and Clinical Significance,** G.A. Jamieson, T.J. Greenwalt, *Editors*

Vol 6: **Prostatic Disease,** H. Marberger, H. Haschek, H.K.A. Schirmer, J.A.C. Colston, E. Witkin, *Editors*

Vol 7: **Blood Pressure, Edema and Proteinuria in Pregnancy,** Emanuel A. Friedman, *Editor*

Vol 8: **Cell Surface Receptors,** Garth L. Nicolson, Michael A. Raftery, Martin Rodbell, C. Fred Fox, *Editors*

Vol 9: **Membranes and Neoplasia: New Approaches and Strategies,** Vincent T. Marchesi, *Editor*

Vol 10: **Diabetes and Other Endocrine Disorders During Pregnancy and in the Newborn,** Maria I. New, Robert H. Fiser, *Editors*

Vol 11: **Clinical Uses of Frozen-Thawed Red Blood Cells,** John A. Griep, *Editor*

Vol 12: **Breast Cancer,** Albert C.W. Montague, Geary L. Stonesifer, Jr., Edward F. Lewison, *Editors*

Vol 13: **The Granulocyte: Function and Clinical Utilization,** Tibor J. Greenwalt, G.A. Jamieson, *Editors*

Vol 14: **Zinc Metabolism: Current Aspects in Health and Disease,** George J. Brewer, Ananda S. Prasad, *Editors*

Vol 15: **Cellular Neurobiology,** Zach Hall, Regis Kelly, C. Fred Fox, *Editors*

Vol 16: **HLA and Malignancy,** Gerald P. Murphy, *Editor*

Vol 17: **Cell Shape and Surface Architecture,** Jean Paul Revel, Ulf Henning, C. Fred Fox, *Editors*

Vol 18: **Tay-Sachs Disease: Screening and Prevention,** Michael M. Kaback, *Editor*

Vol 19: **Blood Substitutes and Plasma Expanders,** G.A. Jamieson, T.J. Greenwalt, *Editors*

Vol 20: **Erythrocyte Membranes: Recent Clinical and Experimental Advances,** Walter C. Kruckeberg, John W. Eaton, George J. Brewer, *Editors*

Vol 21: **The Red Cell,** George J. Brewer, *Editor*

Vol 22: **Molecular Aspects of Membrane Transport,** Dale Oxender, C. Fred Fox, *Editors*

Vol 23: **Cell Surface Carbohydrates and Biological Recognition,** Vincent T. Marchesi, Victor Ginsburg, Phillips W. Robbins, C. Fred Fox, *Editors*

Vol 24: **Twin Research, Proceedings of the Second International Congress on Twin Studies,** Walter E. Nance, *Editor* Published in 3 volumes: Part A: **Psychology and Methodology** Part B: **Biology and Epidemiology** Part C: **Clinical Studies**

Vol 25: **Recent Advances in Clinical Oncology,** Tapan A. Hazra, Michael C. Beachley, *Editors*

Vol 26: **Origin and Natural History of Cell Lines,** Claudio Barigozzi, *Editor*

Vol 27: **Membrane Mechanisms of Drugs of Abuse,** Charles W. Sharp, Leo G. Abood, *Editors*

Vol 28: **The Blood Platelet in Transfusion Therapy,** G.A. Jamieson, Tibor J. Greenwalt, *Editors*

Vol 29: **Biomedical Applications of the Horseshoe Crab (Limulidae),** Elias Cohen, *Editor-in-Chief*

Vol 30: **Normal and Abnormal Red Cell Membranes,** Samuel E. Lux, Vincent T. Marchesi, C. Fred Fox, *Editors*

Vol 31: **Transmembrane Signaling,** Mark Bitensky, R. John Collier, Donald F. Steiner, C. Fred Fox, *Editors*

Vol 32: **Genetic Analysis of Common Diseases: Applications to Predictive Factors in Coronary Disease,** Charles F. Sing, Mark Skolnick, *Editors*

Vol 33: **Prostate Cancer and Hormone Receptors,** Gerald P. Murphy, Avery A. Sandberg, *Editors*

Vol 34: **The Management of Genetic Disorders,** Constantine J. Papadatos, Christos S. Bartsocas, *Editors*

Vol 35: **Antibiotics and Hospitals,** Carlo Grassi, Giuseppe Ostino, *Editors*

Vol 36: **Drug and Chemical Risks to the Fetus, Newborn,** Richard H. Schwarz, Sumner J. Yaffe, *Editors*

Vol 37: **Models for Prostate Cancer,** Gerald P. Murphy, *Editor*

Vol 38: **Ethics, Humanism, and Medicine,** Marc D. Basson, *Editor*

Vol 39: **Neurochemistry and Clinical Neurology,** Leontino Battistin, George Hashim, Abel Lajtha, *Editors*

Vol 40: **Biological Recognition and Assembly,** David S. Eisenberg, James A. Lake, C. Fred Fox, *Editors*

Vol 41: **Tumor Cell Surfaces and Malignancy,** Richard O. Hynes, C. Fred Fox, *Editors*

Vol 42: **Membranes, Receptors, and the Immune Response: 80 Years After Ehrlich's Side Chain Theory,** Edward P. Cohen, Heinz Köhler, *Editors*

Vol 43: **Immunobiology of the Erythrocyte,** S. Gerald Sandler, Jacob Nusbacher, Moses S. Schanfield, *Editors*

Vol 44: **Perinatal Medicine Today,** Bruce K. Young, *Editor*

Vol 45: **Mammalian Genetics and Cancer: The Jackson Laboratory Fiftieth Anniversary Symposium,** Elizabeth S. Russell, *Editor*

Vol 46: **Etiology of Cleft Lip and Cleft Palate,** Michael Melnick, David Bixler, Edward D. Shields, *Editors*

Vol 47: **New Developments With Human and Veterinary Vaccines,** A. Mizrahi, I. Hertman, M.A. Klingberg, A. Kohn, *Editors*

Vol 48: **Cloning of Human Tumor Stem Cells,** Sidney E. Salmon, *Editor*

Vol 49: **Myelin: Chemistry and Biology,** George A. Hashim, *Editor*

Vol 50: **Rights and Responsibilities in Modern Medicine: The Second Volume in a Series on Ethics, Humanism, and Medicine,** Marc D. Basson, *Editor*

Vol 51: **The Function of Red Blood Cells: Erythrocyte Pathobiology,** Donald F. H. Wallach, *Editor*

Vol 52: **Conduction Velocity Distributions: A Population Approach to Electrophysiology of Nerve,** Leslie J. Dorfman, Kenneth L. Cummins, Lary J. Leifer, *Editors*

Vol 53: **Cancer Among Black Populations,** Curtis Mettlin, Gerald P. Murphy, *Editors*

Vol 54: **Connective Tissue Research: Chemistry, Biology, and Physiology,** Zdenek Deyl, Milan Adam, *Editors*

Vol 55: **The Red Cell: Fifth Ann Arbor Conference,** George J. Brewer, *Editor*

Vol 56: **Erythrocyte Membranes 2: Recent Clinical and Experimental Advances,** Walter C. Kruckeberg, John W. Eaton, George J. Brewer, *Editors*

Vol 57: **Progress in Cancer Control,** Curtis Mettlin, Gerald P. Murphy, *Editors*

Vol 58: **The Lymphocyte,** Kenneth W. Sell, William V. Miller, *Editors*

Vol 59: **Eleventh International Congress of Anatomy,** Enrique Acosta Vidrio, *Editor-in-Chief.* Published in 3 volumes: Part A: **Glial and Neuronal Cell Biology,** Sergey Fedoroff, *Editor* Part B: **Advances in the Morphology of Cells and Tissues,** Miguel A. Galina, *Editor* Part C: **Biological Rhythms in Structure and Function,** Heinz von Mayersbach, Lawrence E. Scheving, John E. Pauly, *Editors*

Vol 60: **Advances in Hemoglobin Analysis,** Samir M. Hanash, George J. Brewer, *Editors*

Vol 61: **Nutrition and Child Health: Perspectives for the 1980s,** Reginald C. Tsang, Buford Lee Nichols, Jr., *Editors*

Vol 62: **Pathophysiological Effects of Endotoxins at the Cellular Level,** Jeannine A. Majde, Robert J. Person, *Editors*

Vol 63: **Membrane Transport and Neuroreceptors,** Dale Oxender, Arthur Blume, Ivan Diamond, C. Fred Fox, *Editors*

Vol 64: **Bacteriophage Assembly,** Michael S. DuBow, *Editor*

Vol 65: **Apheresis: Development, Applications, and Collection Procedures,** C. Harold Mielke, Jr., *Editor*

Vol 66: **Control of Cellular Division and Development,** Dennis Cunningham, Eugene Goldwasser, James Watson, C. Fred Fox, *Editors.* Published in 2 volumes.

Vol 67: **Nutrition in the 1980s: Contraints on Our Knowledge,** Nancy Selvey, Philip L. White, *Editors*

Vol 68: **The Role of Peptides and Amino Acids as Neurotransmitters,** J. Barry Lombardini, Alexander D. Kenny, *Editors*

Vol 69: **Twin Research 3, Proceedings of the Third International Congress on Twin Studies,** Ligi Gedda, Paolo Parisi, Walter E. Nance, *Editors.* Published in 3 volumes: Part A: **Twin Biology and Multiple Pregnancy** Part B: **Intelligence, Personality, and Development** Part C: **Epidemiological and Clinical Studies**

Vol 70: **Reproductive Immunology,** Norbert Gleicher, *Editor*

Vol 71: **Psychopharmacology of Clonidine,** Harbans Lal, Stuart Fielding, *Editors*

Vol 72: **Hemophilia and Hemostasis,** Doris Ménaché, D. MacN. Surgenor, Harlan D. Anderson, *Editors*

Vol 73: **Membrane Biophysics: Structure and Function in Epithelia,** Mumtaz A. Dinno, Arthur B. Callahan, *Editors*

Vol 74: **Physiopathology of Endocrine Diseases and Mechanisms of Hormone Action,** Roberto J. Soto, Alejandro De Nicola, Jorge Blaquier, *Editors*

Vol 75: **The Prostatic Cell: Structure and Function,** Gerald P. Murphy, Avery A. Sandberg, James P. Karr, *Editors.* Published in 2 volumes: Part A: **Morphologic, Secretory, and Biochemical Aspects** Part B: **Prolactin, Carcinogenesis, and Clinical Aspects**

Vol 76: **Troubling Problems in Medical Ethics: The Third Volume in a Series on Ethics, Humanism, and Medicine,** Marc D. Basson, Rachel E. Lipson, Doreen L. Ganos, *Editors*

Vol 77: **Nutrition in Health and Disease and International Development: Symposia From the XII International Congress of Nutrition,** Alfred E. Harper, George K. Davis *Editors*

Vol 78: **Female Incontinence,** Norman R. Zinner, Arthur M. Sterling, *Editors*

Vol 79: **Proteins in the Nervous System: Structure and Function,** Bernard Haber, Jose Regino Perez-Polo, Joe Dan Coulter, *Editors*

Vol 80: **Mechanism and Control of Ciliary Movement,** Charles J. Brokaw, Pedro Verdugo, *Editors*

Vol 81: **Physiology and Biology of Horseshoe Crabs: Studies on Normal and Environmentally Stressed Animals,** Joseph Bonaventura, Celia Bonaventura, Shirley Tesh, *Editors*

Vol 82: **Clinical, Structural, and Biochemical Advances in Hereditary Eye Disorders,** Donna L. Daentl, *Editor*

Vol 83: **Issues in Cancer Screening and Communications,** Curtis Mettlin, Gerald P. Murphy, *Editors*

Vol 84: **Progress in Dermatoglyphic Research,** Christos S. Bartsocas, *Editor*

Vol 85: **Embryonic Development,** Max M. Burger, Rudolf Weber, *Editors.* Published in 2 volumes: Part A: **Genetic Aspects** Part B: **Cellular Aspects**

Vol 86: **The Interaction of Acoustical and Electromagnetic Fields With Biological Systems,** Shiro Takashima, Elliot Postow, *Editors*

Vol 87: **Physiopathology of Hypophysial Disturbances and Diseases of Reproduction,** Alejandro De Nicola, Jorge Blaquier, Roberto J. Soto, *Editors*

Vol 88: **Cytapheresis and Plasma Exchange: Clinical Indications,** W.R. Vogler, *Editor*

Vol 89: **Interaction of Platelets and Tumor Cells,** G.A. Jamieson, *Editor*

Vol 90: **Beta-Carbolines and Tetrahydroisoquinolines,** Floyd Bloom, Jack Barchas, Merton Sandler, Earl Usdin, *Organizers*

Vol 91: **Membranes in Growth and Development,** Joseph F. Hoffman, Gerhard H. Giebisch, Liana Bolis, *Editors*

Vol 92: **The Pineal and Its Hormones,** Russel J. Reiter, *Editor*

Vol 93: **Endotoxins and Their Detection With the Limulus Amebocyte Lysate Test,** Stanley W. Watson, Jack Levin, Thomas J. Novitsky, *Editors*

Vol 94: **Animal Models of Inherited Metabolic Diseases,** Robert J. Desnick, Donald F. Patterson, Dante G. Scarpelli, *Editors*

Vol 95: **Gaucher Disease: A Century of Delineation and Research,** Robert J. Desnick, Shimon Gatt, Gregory A. Grabowski, *Editors*

Vol 96: **Mechanisms of Speciation,** Claudio Barigozzi, *Editor*

Vol 97: **Membranes and Genetic Disease,** John R. Sheppard, V. Elving Anderson, John W. Eaton, *Editors*

Vol 98: **Advances in the Pathophysiology, Diagnosis, and Treatment of Sickle Cell Disease,** Roland B. Scott, *Editor*

Vol 99: **Osteosarcoma: New Trends in Diagnosis and Treatment,** Alexander Katznelson, Jacobo Nerubay, *Editors*

Vol 100: **Renal Tumors: Proceedings of the First International Symposium on Kidney Tumors,** René Küss, Gerald P. Murphy, Saad Khoury, James P. Karr, *Editors*

Vol 101: **Factors and Mechanisms Influencing Bone Growth,** Andrew D. Dixon, Bernard G. Sarnat, *Editors*

Vol 102: **Cell Function and Differentiation,** G. Akoyunoglou, A.E. Evangelopoulos, J. Georgatsos, G. Palaiologos, A. Trakatellis, C.P. Tsiganos, *Editors.* Published in 3 volumes. Part A: **Erythroid Differentiation, Hormone-Gene Interaction, Glycoconjugates, Liposomes, Cell Growth, and Cell-Cell Interaction.** Part B: **Biogenesis of Energy Transducing Membranes and Membrane and Protein Energetics.** Part C: **Enzyme Structure—Mechanism, Metabolic Regulations, and Phosphorylation-Dephosphorylation Processes**

Vol 103: **Human Genetics,** Batsheva Bonné-Tamir, *Editor,* Tirza Cohen, Richard M. Goodman, *Associate Editors.* Published in 2 volumes. Part A: **The Unfolding Genome.** Part B: **Medical Aspects**

Vol 104: **Skeletal Dysplasias,** C.J. Papadatos, C.S. Bartsocas, *Editors*

Vol 105: **Polyomaviruses and Human Neurological Diseases,** John L. Sever, David L. Madden, *Editors*

Vol 106: **Therapeutic Apheresis and Plasma Perfusion,** Richard S.A. Tindall, *Editor*

Vol 107: **Biomedical Thermology,** Michel Gautherie, Ernest Albert, *Editors*

Vol 108: **Massive Transfusion in Surgery and Trauma,** John A. Collins, Kris Murawski, A. William Shafer, *Editors*

Vol 109: **Mutagens in Our Environment,** Marja Sorsa, Harri Vainio, *Editors*

Vol 110: **Limb Development and Regeneration.** Published in 2 volumes. **Part A,** John F. Fallon, Arnold I. Caplan, *Editors.* **Part B,** Robert O. Kelley, Paul F. Goetinck, Jeffrey A. MacCabe, *Editors*

Vol 111: **Molecular and Cellular Aspects of Shock and Trauma,** Allan M. Lefer, William Schumer, *Editors*

Vol 112: **Recent Advances in Fertility Research,** Thomas G. Muldoon, Virendra B. Mahesh, Bautista Pérez-Ballester, *Editors.* Published in two volumes. Part A: **Developments in Reproductive Endocrinology.** Part B: **Developments in the Management of Reproductive Disorders**

Vol 113: **The S-Potential,** Boris D. Drujan, Miguel Laufer, *Editors*

Vol 114: **Enzymology of Carbonyl Metabolism: Aldehyde Dehydrogenase and Aldo/Keto Reductase,** Henry Weiner, Bendicht Wermuth, *Editors*